NURSING PROCESS HANDBOOK

NURSING PROCESS HANDBOOK

Patricia W. Hickey, R.N., B.S.N., P.H.N., M.N.

Assistant Professor
Medical-Surgical Nursing
Cypress Community College
Cypress, California

with **5** *illustrations*

The C. V. Mosby Company

ST. LOUIS • PHILADELPHIA •
BALTIMORE • TORONTO   1990

Mosby

Editor: Nancy L. Coon
Developmental editor: Susan R. Epstein
Project manager: Patricia Tannian
Production editor: John Casey
Book and cover design: Gail Morey Hudson

Copyright © 1990 by The C.V. Mosby Company

Printed in the United States of America

The C.V. Mosby Company
11830 Westline Industrial Drive, St. Louis, Missouri 63146

Library of Congress Cataloging in Publication Data

Hickey, Patricia W.
    Nursing process handbook/Patricia W. Hickey.
      p.   cm.
    Includes bibliographies and index.
ISBN 0-8016-6041-6
    1. Nursing—Handbooks, manuals, etc. I. Title.
    [DNLM: 1. Nursing Process.   WY 100 H628n]
RT51.H48 1990
610.73—dc20
DNLM/DLC
for Library of Congress   89–8298
ISBN 0-8016-6041-6   CIP

GW/RRD/RRD 9 8 7 6 5 4 3 2 1

Preface

This is a book about caring—professional caring, nursing caring. As long as there have been people, there has been nursing: people taking care of others. This human tradition is instinctive and untrained; it is the natural art of nursing: human caring for humans.

Professional nursing, which is both an art and a science, evolved from those early practitioners. Florence Nightingale is credited with establishing nursing as a trained profession. Since those early days of the profession, nursing has increasingly acquired a more scientific aspect. Expanding technology has demanded that nurses become technologically proficient. Consumer health awareness and economic conditions have mandated increased nursing efficiency.

The nursing profession has continually

met these challenges. Nursing training has changed; it has become formalized and regulated education. Nursing practice has undergone a revolution. From artful caring, it has emerged into a dynamic collaborative profession having its own body of specialized scientific knowledge and standards of practice. It has its own framework for practice that identifies it as a profession: the nursing process.

The nursing process is the tool by which nurses continue the human tradition of caring. It is the modern adaptation of an evolving profession to age-old needs. It enables the nurse to use scientific advances, not to make nursing cold and impersonally scientific, but rather to provide quality, personalized human caring.

Contents

1

Nursing Process
AN OVERVIEW

- **Definition**
- **Necessity**
- **Advantages**

Nurses work in a wide variety of settings, from acute care hospitals to outpatient clinics to individually owned health-care businesses. The conditions and concerns they deal with are even more diverse, from conception to death and from illness to health. In caring for people of all ages and cultures, nurses employ a breadth of skills that spans the specialties.

Nursing specialties appear to share few things in common. Each specialty, whether it be intensive care, rehabilitation, home health, obstetrics, or psychiatry, has its own characteristics and particular expertise. However, a common thread is woven through all of this diversity in nursing: the nursing process. Despite the vast array of knowledge and skills needed for any area of nursing, every nurse must know and practice the *process of nursing*. This process is not *what* the nurse does, but it is the *method* by which the nurse practices.

DESCRIPTION

The nursing process is a systematic method by which nurses plan and provide care for clients. This involves a problem-solving approach that enables the nurse to identify client problems and needs and to plan, deliver, and evaluate nursing care in an orderly, scientific manner. The framework of the nursing process enables the nurse to focus on client needs and to apply the broad base of nursing knowledge in an organized fashion. Figure 1 shows the interrelationships of the five sequential steps in the nursing process.

Assessment, the first step of the process, entails the collection of physiologic, developmental, psychologic, cognitive, social, and spiritual information in an organized for-

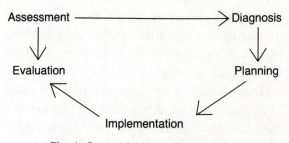

Fig. 1. *Steps of the nursing process.*

mat. Methods of data collection include the interview, physical examination, observation, consultation, and chart research. The assessment phase of the nursing process yields facts about the client and significant others; these are then sorted and grouped into categories of nursing concerns. These clusters of data form the basis for problem identification.

Diagnosis is the analysis of the data that have been gathered and organized. Data are analyzed from a nursing perspective and result in formal statements of the client's actual and potential health-related problems. Nursing diagnoses give the nurse focus and direction in planning goal-directed care.

Planning requires setting goals and selecting interventions. Based on the identified problems the nurse and client together plan how to resolve each problem in the most effective manner.

Implementation involves putting the care plan into action. After the environment, supplies, and client are prepared, interventions are carried out as planned.

Evaluation is the last and crucial step of the process. Established goals are reviewed in terms of client accomplishment. If the goals have been met, the process is terminated. If the goals have not been met, the process is reactivated in sequence, with each step evaluated and revised consecutively.

BENEFITS

The nursing process has benefits for the client, nurse, and nursing as a profession.

The client

The client reaps five benefits when the nursing process is used. First, the client becomes an active participant in health care. Since every step of the process requires client input, a partnership is formed with the nurse and unnecessary client dependence is prevented. Continuous client involvement encourages trust and motivation.

Second, client input also ensures an individualized care plan. Individual needs and responses are considered at every step.

Third, the client receives high-quality, comprehensive care. The nursing process is dynamic and provides for ongoing assessment and care plan revision in response to changing needs. This ensures ongoing identification of and provision for client needs.

Fourth, the focus of care is consistent. Communication and documentation at every step coordinate care delivery. When all team members work together, continuity of care results.

Fifth, the nursing process provides cost-effective client care. The efficiency of identifying individual problems and needs and providing high-quality continuity of care reduces the length of treatment. Treatment costs are reduced, and eventually cost reduction is reflected in insurance premiums.

The nurse

The systematic format of the nursing process, with its focus on the client's re-

sponse to illness, has advantages and re-
wards for the individual nurse providing
care. The first advantage the nurse may no-
tice is easier routine nursing care. Because
client problems have been identified and a
care plan formulated, the nurse does not
have to "reinvent the wheel" every day. Providing care becomes a matter of ongoing
assessment, implementation, and evaluation
as planned. The nurse's time and energy can
be spent on problem resolution.

The nurse also discovers enhanced cre-
ativity. The structured framework of the
nursing process encourages professional
growth and creative approaches to problem
solving. Collaboration at each step of the
process provides opportunities for fresh
ideas. Additional benefits stemming from
collaboration are a sense of community and
a feeling of belonging.

Finally the nurse experiences increased
job satisfaction. Frustration and burnout,
which frequently result from a lack of organization, are prevented. The care plan
provides specific direction; the nurse is
aware of current client problems and what
needs to be accomplished. As the care plan
is implemented and evaluated, the nurse ob-

tains objective evidence of client improvement. This sense of organization, direction, and effectiveness is very rewarding to the nurse.

Nursing profession

The nursing process defines nursing's professional role to the nurse, society, and other health-care professions. At the same time it ensures the professional practice of nursing.

Defining nursing's role

Nursing, as stated by the American Nurses' Association (ANA), is dedicated to the diagnosis and treatment of client problems that arise as a result of an illness. In other words the concern of nursing is not the medical condition or treatment but the client's actual or potential unhealthful response to the illness. The nursing process keeps nursing attention focused on these human responses.

Through the use of the nursing process, this nursing perspective becomes apparent to the client. The client, participating in each step of the process, is aware of the nurse's role in providing health care. Thus the client and society come to view nursing as a distinct profession.

Through practice and documentation the nursing process differentiates nursing from other professions. For instance, medicine is concerned with the client's illness and treatment. Radiology deals with the visualization of the disease process. Physical therapy concentrates on the maintenance and restoration of movement. Nursing's concern is for the client's well-being; the nurse's goal is the restoration of the client's ability to complete the activities of daily living in a healthful manner. Differences in perspective and approach characterize each profession; the combination of the perspectives and approaches provides comprehensive client care.

Although nursing is distinct from other health-care professions, it also works with them in providing total client care. This collaborative approach requires independent, interdependent, and dependent nursing functions.

The *independent* functions of nursing define nursing as a profession and include those activities that nurses are educated and licensed to perform autonomously. The five steps of the nursing process, which diagnose and treat the human responses to illness, are defined by the ANA as the exclusive domain of professional nursing. These actions are authorized by the nursing license. All nursing diagnoses are examples of independent nursing functions, since they identify concerns that are solely those of the nursing profession.

The *interdependent* functions of nursing involve collaboration with other health-oriented professions. Although needing nursing expertise, these activities are performed in conjunction with other professions and receive their authority for initiation from a physician's order. Managing care of a nasogastric tube is an example of an interdependent function. Insertion of the tube requires a medical order, but its maintenance is a nursing responsibility.

Dependent functions are nursing actions directly implementing medical orders. They require technical nursing knowledge and skill but may be performed only on a physician's explicit order. Administration of medications is an example of a dependent nursing action. The physician prescribes; the nurse administers the medication as prescribed and monitors effects and side effects. Whenever implementing medical orders the nurse must simultaneously exercise the independent functions of assessment and evaluation.

When writing the care plan the nurse must be careful to include all three levels of functions, as necessitated by the client's needs. By keeping in mind the role of nursing in the overall care plan, the nurse maintains a sense of nursing identity, developing self-awareness as a nurse, with skills, knowledge, and a perspective unique to nursing. Thus identifying the role of nursing defines nursing as a profession.

Ensuring professional practice

The ANA has published eight standards of practice for professional nurses. State nurse practice acts mandate these same criteria and make nurses legally accountable for them. The nursing process encompasses these standards.

The professional and legal codes hold nurses accountable for each step of the nursing process and its documentation. Nurses are held accountable for the accurate assessment of client information, the diagnosis of unhealthful responses based on the data, the establishment of a prioritized care plan relevant to the nursing diagnoses, the skilled implementation of the nursing care plan, the evaluation of the effectiveness of nursing care, and the complete and accurate documentation of each step. Careful implementation of every step of the process prevents malpractice, negligence, or both, and ensures the maintenance of quality care in the nursing practice.

SUMMARY

The nursing process is composed of five steps (assessment, diagnosis, planning, implementation, and evaluation) by which nurses organize the practice of nursing. These steps, sequential and closely interrelated, serve as a systematic process that protects and benefits the client, the individual nurse, and the nursing profession.

When the nursing process is used, clients become actively involved in all phases of their care. This makes care highly individualized and responsive to the client's particular needs. The result is high-quality, comprehensive, cost-effective continuity of care.

The individual nurse benefits from the structured approach, with economy of time and energies, enhanced professional growth, a sense of profession, and increased job satisfaction.

The nursing profession is advanced through the definition of nursing's unique role in overall client care. The nursing process provides the means by which nurses fulfill both professional and legal responsibilities, for which they are accountable.

BIBLIOGRAPHY

American Nurses' Association: Standards of nursing practice, Kansas City, Mo, 1973, The Association.

American Nurses' Association: Nursing: a social policy statement, Kansas City, Mo, 1980, The Association.

Andersen JE and Briggs LL: Nursing diagnosis: a study of quality and supportive evidence, Image 20:141, 1988.

Kozier B and Erb G: Fundamentals of nursing: concepts and procedures, ed 3, Menlo Park, Calif, 1987, Addison-Wesley Publishing Co, Inc.

Luckman J and Sorensen DC: Medical-surgical nursing: a psychophysiologic approach, ed 3, Philadelphia, 1987, WB Saunders Co.

Phipps WJ, Long BC, and Woods NF: Medical-surgical nursing: concepts and clinical practice, ed 3, St Louis, 1987, The CV Mosby Co.

Potter PA and Perry AG: Fundamentals of nursing: concepts, process, and practice, ed 2, St Louis, 1989, The CV Mosby Co.

Tamparong F: Personal communication, November 13, 1986.

2
Assessment

- Data collection
- Data sorting
- Data documentation

The nursing process begins with a thorough assessment of the client. The nurse sorts and analyzes the collected data and then formulates the care plan. Assessment allows the nurse to individualize the care plan to the particular client.

The assessment phase of the nursing process includes (1) collecting the data in a systematic manner, (2) sorting and organizing the data, and (3) documenting the data in an organized format.

DATA COLLECTION

Client assessment begins on admission and continues until discharge. The admission assessment establishes a baseline for problem identification. Ongoing assessments monitor the client's status in regard to identified problems and new complications.

When assessing a client it is best if the nurse uses a methodic approach to ensure that no significant information is overlooked. This deliberate approach to client assessment need not be impersonal. By demonstrating genuine interest in and concern for the client the nurse can achieve personalized caring within the structured format. Most clients find reassurance and security in knowing that they are being thoroughly assessed and carefully treated.

Client information is organized into subjective and objective data. *Subjective data* are obtained during the client interview. This information includes the client's perspective, feelings, thoughts, and expectations, which are things that cannot be directly observed and can be discovered only by asking questions. Because subjective data are the client's perspective regarding the illness and general health status, these are essential to a complete data base.

Objective data are information including

all those things about the client that can be directly observed by others. These facts about the client's condition and behavior complete the data base and provide concrete and unbiased information from an impartial observer's perspective.

It is recommended that for the sake of efficiency the nurse use a "branching" technique during each phase of data collection. "Branching" means that the nurse further investigates those areas of the assessment in which a dysfunction or abnormality appears to exist and abbreviates the assessment in those areas in which no problem is apparent.

Subjective data: the client interview

The first step in establishing a data base is to collect subjective information by interviewing the client. By placing the interview first the nurse has an opportunity to do the following:

1. Establish a therapeutic relationship with the client
2. Introduce the client to the facility in a nonthreatening manner
3. Gain insight into the client's concerns and worries

4. Obtain cues as to which of the remaining parts of the data collection
phase require in-depth investigation
(branching)

Client interviews are composed of an introduction, a body, and a conclusion. During the introductory phase the nurse in-
troduces herself or himself by name and
position and states the purpose of the interview. The nurse then assures the client
that all information will be kept confiden-
tial. These courtesies allay client anxieties
about divulging personal information to a
stranger and enlist the client as a partner in
health-care management. The body of the
interview is designed to gather as much information as possible pertinent to the
client's health status. It should be focused,
orderly, and conducted in an unhurried
manner. In concluding the interview the
nurse summarizes the important points and
asks the client if the summary is accurate.
Validation of the interview is essential, since
it allows the client to clarify or add information.

The admission, or initial, interview is
normally the most extensive of all interviews. Major topics to be covered include

demographic data, current illness, and health history.

Demographic data, as specified by the facility, are collected first. Since this information is the least personal, it helps to initiate development of the therapeutic relationship and to ease transition into the body of the interview.

In the body of the interview the current illness and health history are investigated systematically. Areas to be assessed include the following:

1. The problem requiring medical attention and related medical history
2. Symptoms, including onset, duration, frequency, and intensity
3. Contributing factors to the problem, that is, what makes it worse and what makes it better
4. How the client has been treating the problem, including what works and what does not work
5. How the physician has been treating the problem, including the effects and side effects of the treatment
6. The client's perception of the illness, that is, personal feelings and expectations

7. Other health problems, current and previous
8. Support systems, social and environmental assets and deficits

Ongoing, or continuing, interviews need not be so extensive; they should be updates on the client's status and more focused toward changes in problems previously identified, as well as any new developments. Many aspects of the admission interview, such as the demographic data, can be omitted, since these have been previously documented and can be reviewed on the chart if necessary. Ongoing interviews should concentrate on maintaining the therapeutic relationship, monitoring the client's subjective progress or lack of progress, and identifying any new concerns or client needs. Whereas the admission interview centers on problem identification, the continuing interview focuses more on evaluation and prevention.

If the client is hospitalized, the nurse caring for the client should conduct a brief ongoing interview at the beginning of each shift to validate any changes in status. In outpatient situations the nurse should ask the client for health status updates at every visit.

General guidelines for interviewing

The manner in which the interview is conducted is just as important as the questions asked. Attention to environmental aspects and client comfort, as well as communication techniques, ensures a successful interview.

Environmental aspects include providing for privacy and eliminating distractions, unnecessary noise, and interruptions. The client is much more likely to be candid if the interview is conducted privately, out of earshot of other clients, visitors, and staff. Privacy and quiet may be provided by going to an unoccupied room or drawing the curtains around the bed. Noise and distractions can be reduced by requesting that the television and radio remain off during the interview. Timing is important in avoiding interruptions. If possible, a 15- to 30-minute time period should be set aside when no other activities are planned. The client should be made to feel relaxed and unhurried.

Before beginning, the client should be made comfortable. This includes adequate light, warmth, and positioning. The client should be sitting as upright as possible to facilitate eye contact. During the interview the nurse should be alert to signs of client discomfort or tiring.

Good communication starts with a non-judgmental, interested, and caring attitude. This is more readily conveyed nonverbally if the nurse and client are at approximately the same eye level. The nurse should sit facing the client whenever possible. Throughout the interview a variety of communication techniques should be used. Initially, open questions prevent stalls and provide the opportunity for the client to indicate major concerns. When more specific information about a topic is needed, closed questions serve best. "Why" questions are to be avoided because they are often unanswerable and sometimes make the client defensive. Conducting the interview by only asking questions may make the client feel like a subject of interrogation. Other communication techniques, such as reflecting, making observations, and clarifying, should be interspersed throughout the interview to encourage the exchange of information. If the client is very talkative, the nurse may need to refocus the interview when the client strays from the topic. Summarization and validation are always used when concluding an interview. Active listening is imperative during the entire interview; it makes the nurse alert to unspoken clues and reinforces the therapeutic relationship.

Objective data

The remainder of the data collection process is concerned with obtaining observable information that is undistorted by the client's perceptions. Objective data are collected from the physical assessment, observation of client behavior, and other sources.

The physical assessment

Collection of objective data begins with the physical assessment. As with the interview, it is best to begin the physical assessment in a nonthreatening manner. This can be accomplished by starting with the familiar procedure of taking vital signs.

The actual hands-on physical assessment should be conducted so that the client's anxiety is not aroused. The nurse should explain each step and continue talking to the client throughout, explaining and asking about specific function and discomfort. It is also important to protect the client's privacy and dignity and to make sure she or he is warm; uncover and cover each body part in turn.

The physical assessment should proceed in an orderly sequence, using the four techniques of inspection, auscultation, palpation, and percussion as appropriate. The nurse may select whichever examination format is most comfortable. The most common formats are (1) the head-to-toe (cephalocaudal) approach, (2) the systems method, and (3) the client-needs format. Examples of each assessment approach are given in Appendix A.

In the *head-to-toe* assessment the nurse examines the client in a physically consecutive manner, that is, each body part is examined for structure and function, starting with the head and working down the trunk and extremities in an orderly fashion. Major advantages of this method include the ease of remembering the examination's sequence and the unlikelihood of overlooking a body part. The main disadvantage is the need for extensive sorting and organizing of data, since, for instance, the skin covers the entire body.

The *systems* assessment parallels the medical model in that the nurse examines the body by organic functional systems, such as respiratory, cardiac, and vascular. The main advantage of this approach is that the data are already organized according to the physician's format of physical dysfunction. Disadvantages include the need for considerable data reorganization and, especially in the beginning, the relative ease of skipping a body system and thus missing pertinent data.

The *client-needs* assessment involves examining the client from a biopsychosocial functional approach and it includes analyzing biologic, developmental, psychologic, cultural, social, and religious factors. Assessing client needs includes, for example, assessing the needs for nutrition and elimination. Advantages of this method include the gathering and organization of data according to the nursing perspective. Disadvantages are that these categories are not always exclusive of each other and therefore may be difficult to analyze, and that a thorough understanding of nursing's role, such as that specified in a nursing model, is needed to carry out a comprehensive assessment when using this approach.

If the nurse is using a *nursing model,* the conceptual framework of the model guides the approach and organization of the assessment. For instance, Johnson's model views the client in terms of behavioral subsystems, whereas Orem's model examines the client for self-care capabilities and deficits. The advantages of using a nursing model include the clear focusing of data toward a particular nursing perspective and the clear identification of nursing's role in client care. The major disadvantage of this approach is that the rest of the health-care team may not be familiar with the model and its particular viewpoint and terminology.

Whichever physical assessment method the nurse uses, all essential areas of concern need to be examined. The nurse may verify this by running through a mental checklist of the examination's sequence so nothing will be omitted.

The admission physical assessment is the longest and most extensive of assessments because it establishes a baseline of both normal and abnormal findings. The ongoing physical assessment is briefer, focusing on those areas in which a dysfunction or abnormality was initially found and on those areas in which there was an initial assessment of potential dysfunction. As with the interview, familiarity with the client and previously documented information quickens and abbreviates the process.

Observation of behavior

During both the interview and the physical assessment, the nurse should observe the client's behavior for level of function, consistency, and congruency. This information adds greater depth to the objective data base.

The *level of function* includes physical, developmental, psychologic, and social aspects. Observation of the level of function differs from the interview in that this is what the nurse *sees* the client doing, rather than what the client *states* can be performed. Level of function differs from the physical assessment in that this is the degree of function at which the client is *operating*, rather than the *greatest extent* of function present determined by the hands-on assessment.

Consistency refers to the degree to which the client operates at the same level of functioning (physical, developmental, psychologic, and social) throughout the assessment and day by day. Any inconsistency is worthy of further investigation.

Congruency is the matching or agreement between two or more things. The client's statements should match mood and behavior. The subjective data (the client's statements) and the objective data (the physical assessment, the client's behavior, and the medical record) should be in general agreement. Incongruencies indicate the need for further data collection.

Other sources

To this point, data have been collected only from the client. Other valuable sources of information include (1) the family or significant others, (2) the health-care team, and (3) the client's medical record. These resources can add an extra dimension to the fund of knowledge about the client by supplying unsuspected bits of information and a third party's insight.

Significant others know the client from a point of view unavailable to the health-care team. They frequently are able to provide background information essential to understanding the client's situation and responses.

The *health-care team* includes the physician, other nurses, and the ancillary staff. They can be invaluable in giving insights into client behavior and needs.

The *medical record* provides pertinent data about the client's medical history, diagnostic studies, and the physician's proposed treatment plan. The nurse should use the chart not only as a resource for additional information, but also as a tool for checking the consistency and congruency of her or his own observations. Nursing notes, frequently overlooked, are an excellent means for accomplishing this latter function.

SORTING THE DATA

Once the subjective and objective data have been collected from all of the above areas, the nurse needs to organize the information into meaningful and usable clusters, keeping in mind nursing's unique point of view, that is, the client's response to illness. The nurse bases this sorting of data on professional knowledge.

If the nurse has been trained to use a nursing model (Johnson, Rogers, Orem, and others), the data are sorted according to the designated categories. These categories give the data meaning from the nursing model's point of view. If the nurse is not using a specific nursing model, a framework is selected to organize the data. This framework can be the same as that used for conducting the physical assessment, that is, sorting by anatomy, by organic systemic function, or by client needs. Each of these approaches can be adapted to nursing's perspective of caring for the client's unhealthful response to the illness or condition.

Sorting data by anatomy

When sorting data by anatomy the nurse separates the data according to body part. This type of organization places the nurse's focus on that type of anatomic assistance that the client needs to recover. An example of sorted anatomic data follows:

Head	Skin color dusky with circumoral cyanosis; pursed-lip breathing
Chest	Barrel shaped, suprasternal retrac-

tions; uses accessory muscles for respiration; respiratory rate 28; crackles and wheezes throughout lung fields

Sorting data by organic system function

Sorting data by organic system function involves separating and organizing in a manner similar to that of the physician. This format directs the nurse's attention to those functions needing support and assistance for recovery. One example of system sorting is the following:

Respiratory   Respirations 28, shallow and irregular; pursed-lip breathing; circumoral cyanosis; barrel-shaped chest; suprasternal retractions; crackles and wheezes throughout lung fields; arterial blood gases (ABGs) indicate respiratory acidosis; history of chronic obstructive pulmonary disease (COPD) for 5 years

Cardiac   Heart rate 96 and irregular; radiograph reveals enlarged cardiac silhouette; history of congestive heart failure (CHF) for 3 years

Sorting data by client needs

Sorting data by client needs leads directly to nursing diagnoses. This sytem may initially be the most difficult for the beginning nurse, unless the nurse uses a nursing model. However, no matter what format is used to gather information, the data can be sorted by client needs, using the functional health patterns identified by Marjory Gordon (1982) or those included in any nursing model. Gordon lists the following eleven need categories:

1. Health perception–health management
2. Nutrition-metabolic
3. Elimination
4. Activity-exercise
5. Sleep-rest
6. Cognitive-perceptual
7. Self-perception–self-concept
8. Role-relationship
9. Sexuality-reproductive
10. Coping–stress tolerance
11. Value-belief

The following is an example of sorting data by client needs:

Health management	Uses oxygen at home; takes bronchodilators when he remembers
Activity-exercise	Becomes dyspneic and short of breath (SOB) upon ambulation; unable to perform activities of daily living (ADLs) without frequent rest periods
Sleep-rest	Three-pillow orthopnea; frequent episodes of nocturnal paroxysmal dyspnea

DOCUMENTING THE DATA

Two of the most important things to remember about recording client data are thoroughness and factualness. Documentation is the only lasting remainder of a complete assessment. If an item is not recorded, that information is lost and unavailable to anyone researching the chart. If specific information is not given, the reader is left with general impressions because of the lack of factual information.

Thoroughness in data documentation is essential for two reasons: (1) all data pertinent to the client's status is included, and (2) the observation and recording of the client's status is legally a professional responsibility.

The first reason for thoroughness refers to the client's benefit, ensuring that full information is available to all those caring for the client's needs. Even information that does not seem particularly relevant should be recorded. It may become important later, serving as baseline data for a change in status. A general rule of thumb: *if it was assessed, it should be recorded.*

The second reason for thoroughness concerns the nurse's professional proficiency and protection of the nursing license. The nurse practice acts in all states and the ANA Policy Statement (1980) mandate accurate data collection and recording as independent functions essential to the role of the professional nurse. Thorough documentation visibly demonstrates professional competence and provides protection of the license by demonstrating that professional responsibilities were met. The following example may seem obvious, but it occurs frequently in nurses' charting:

Incorrect	Voiding qs
Correct	Voiding without difficulty; urine straw-colored, clear, slight am-

> monia odor, intake and output
> (I & O) in balance

In the above example the correct documentation indicates no specific problem at this time, but it provides an accurate picture for later reference. The incorrect example provides almost no information; in fact it is uncertain whether that part of the assessment was actually conducted.

Being *factual* is easy once the habit is formed. The basic rule is to record what is *observed*. When recording data, attention should be paid to facts, and efforts should be made to be as descriptive as possible. What is heard, seen, felt, and smelled should be reported exactly. It is important not to generalize or to jump to conclusions. Conclusions about observations eventually become nursing diagnoses.

Nurses are so accustomed to gathering data and quickly making judgments that this fundamental principle of data documentation (that is, to avoid jumping to conclusions) is often violated. Because of a great familiarity with the constellation of signs and symptoms accompanying a specific problem, the nurse often immediately assumes the existence of that problem. The assumption is charted as data, and the actual facts are lost. If discovering that this approach was used, the nurse should reevaluate and ask, "what actual things did I observe to make me arrive at that conclusion?" All facts should be obtained and recorded before generalizations are made. Clustering the data too soon leads to faulty diagnoses. The following example illustrates a common error in generalization.

Incorrect	Angry
Correct	Refused medication; shouted loudly when offered medication; threw pillow across room; body in hunched position in bed

Here the incorrect example probably indicates the problem correctly, but it provides no baseline facts by which to evaluate change. The correct documentation lists observable behaviors that can be compared with later behavior.

SUMMARY

Data collection and documentation are the foundations for the care plan. The care plan therefore can be only as good as the data on which it is based.

When assessing the client the nurse

should keep an organizational format in mind. This ensures that no critical parts are missed. Data should be gathered from a variety of sources: the client interview and physical assessment, observation of client behavior, and other sources, such as the client's significant others, the health-care team, and the medical record. A well-rounded assessment ensures a well-balanced view of the client.

After the data have been collected the nurse needs to sort and organize the information into related groups. This analysis and synthesis of data are the preparatory steps toward making a nursing diagnosis.

The assessed data should be documented thoroughly and factually, with observations described in measurable terms. Major normal and abnormal findings should be included in each category that was assessed. If some pertinent data were not collected, the care plan will be insufficient to meet the client's needs. If all pertinent data were collected but not well documented, the care plan will contain elements that are not justified in the medical record. Accuracy and thoroughness in the assessment stage are essential to good care planning.

NURSING CARE PLAN

Discharge Goal:

ASSESSMENT	NURSING DIAGNOSIS
Subjective data Interview	

Objective data
  Physical examination
  Health record
  Observation of be-
    havior
  Other sources	

Data organization	

EXPECTED OUTCOMES   INTERVENTIONS   EVALUATION

BIBLIOGRAPHY

American Nurses' Association: Nursing: a social policy statement, Kansas City, Mo, 1980, The Association.

Auger JR: Behavioral systems and nursing, Englewood Cliffs, NJ, 1976, Prentice Hall.

Bates B: Physical examination and history taking, ed 4, Philadelphia, 1987, JB Lippincott Co.

Carpenito LJ: Handbook of nursing diagnosis, ed 2, Philadelphia, 1987, JB Lippincott Co.

Carter FM: Psychosocial nursing: theory and practice in hospital and community mental health, ed 3, New York, 1981, Macmillan Publishing Co.

Gordon M: Nursing diagnosis: process and application, New York, 1987, McGraw-Hill, Inc.

Ivey AE: Intentional interviewing and counseling: facilitating client development, ed 2, Pacific Grove, Calif, 1988, Brooks/Cole Publishing Co.

Nursing85 Books: Practices, Springhouse, Pa, 1985, Springhouse Corp.

Orem DE: Nursing: concepts of practice, ed 3, New York, 1985, McGraw-Hill, Inc.

Riehl JP and Roy C: Conceptual models for nursing practice, ed 2, New York, 1980, Appleton & Lange.

Roy C: Introduction to nursing: an adaptation model, Englewood Cliffs, NJ, 1976, Prentice Hall.

3
Diagnosis

- *Data analysis*
- *Problem identification*
- *Format*
- *Prioritization*
- *Documentation*

The second step in the nursing process is the diagnostic statement, which is the result of a careful analysis of all the data collected from the interview, physical assessment, and chart review. During the assessment phase, as previously mentioned, the data are gathered and sorted into related topics. In the diagnostic phase the nurse, using professional knowledge as a guide, analyzes the information to make a judgment. The nurse's specialized education provides the basis and the focus for this analysis. The resulting judgment is written as a nursing diagnosis.

A nursing diagnosis is a statement of the client's actual or potential unhealthful response to an unhealthful condition or illness. A closer look at each portion of this definition follows.

Term	Definition
Nursing	Conducted by the nurse; within the domain of nursing practice, for which the nurse is educationally and legally responsible; distinct from medicine
Diagnosis	A statement defining or identifying a problem; the result of data analysis
Statement	A declaration or proposition that offers a judgment or fact; consists of two parts: problem and etiology
Client's	Referring to the client, the person with the condition or illness; distinct from nursing or medicine
Actual	A problem that currently exists and that has been clinically validated
Potential	A problem that is imminent or likely to occur; usually preventable
Unhealthful	That which does not promote well-being; maladaptive
Response	A reaction to a causative factor; in this case the resulting effects that the client experiences secondary to the unhealthful condition or disease

Condition/ illness	Those physical, mental, or psychologic ailments that are diagnosed by the physician

Both the nurses's role and the criteria for writing nursing diagnoses can be identified by examining each portion of the definition.

Nurse's role

Nursing diagnoses define client problems from a nursing perspective and are part of the independent role of nursing. Once written, they become the direct responsibility of the nurse, who must activate the entire sequence of the nursing process to resolve the problem.

Because the nursing diagnosis deals with the *client's response* to an illness or condition rather than the ailment itself, it clearly distinguishes the nurse's role from that of the physician. It helps the nurse to focus on nursing's independent role and to refrain from practicing medicine. It also keeps attention focused on those concerns that the nurse is educationally and legally qualified to treat. The following is an example of this differentiation.

Medical	**Nursing**
Diagnosis	
COPD	Impaired gas exchange related to tenacious mucous secretions
Treatment	
O$_2$, medication, etc.	Paced activity, breathing techniques, etc.

Criteria for writing a nursing diagnosis

It is becoming more important, legally and professionally, for nurses to write accurate diagnoses. To verify that a nursing diagnosis is appropriate, the following four criteria must be met:

1. The problem is identified as a response to an illness.
2. Identification of the problem requires professional analysis of assessed client data.
3. The nurse is legally and educationally capable of diagnosing the problem.
4. The necessary interventions for problem resolution are legally within the scope of nursing to order and implement.

Included after each criterion here are examples of correct and incorrect nursing diagnoses, which illustrate one of the above criteria, as they might be written for a client with the medical diagnosis of arthritis.

1. The problem is identified as a response to an illness.
   a. *Incorrect nursing diagnosis*—Impaired home maintenance management related to lack of home help
   b. *Correct nursing diagnosis*—Impaired home maintenance management related to joint stiffness

In this example the incorrect diagnosis indicates a problem originating in an area unrelated to an illness. The correct diagnosis, on the other hand, identifies the physical consequences of arthritis that are causing the problem in maintaining home management.

2. Identification of the problem requires professional analysis of assessed client data.
   a. *Incorrect nursing diagnosis*—Upset stomach related to aspirin ingestion
   b. *Correct nursing diagnosis*—Alteration in nutrition, less than body requirements

> related to gastrointestinal side effects
> of aspirin therapy

Here the incorrect diagnosis states only readily apparent facts; it required no professional expertise to formulate, since it is generally understood that aspirin can upset the stomach. The correct version is based on the nurse's understanding of aspirin ingestion, which often causes gastrointestinal discomfort and results in decreased nutritional intake.

3. The nurse is legally and educationally capable of diagnosing the problem.
   a. *Incorrect nursing diagnosis*—Alteration in comfort, chronic pain related to arthritis
   b. *Correct nursing diagnosis*—Alteration in comfort, chronic pain related to overuse of inflamed joints; *or,* Alteration in comfort, chronic pain related to effects of arthritis

The etiology of the incorrect diagnosis is a restatement of the medical diagnosis. Since the nurse is not educationally prepared to diagnose medical problems, the statement is legally inadvisable. The correct diagnoses use etiologies within the scope of nursing practice. The nurse is competent to deal with the *effects of* a medical diagnosis. The first correct nursing diagnosis, which is the better of the two, identifies which particular effect is the major source of the chronic pain.

4. The necessary interventions for problem resolution are legally within the scope of the nursing profession to order and implement.
   a. *Incorrect nursing diagnosis* — Ineffective individual coping related to chronic illness
   b. *Correct nursing diagnosis* — Ineffective individual coping related to noncompliance with treatment regimen

As discussed in Chapter 4, the nurse plans interventions toward the etiology of the problem. In the incorrect version of the diagnosis the nurse cannot independently order and implement any interventions to resolve the chronic illness. Conversely, in the correct statement, it is within the nurse's independent role to deal with noncompliant responses.

If the four criteria are met, the nursing diagnosis is appropriate and serves to ensure maintenance of legal and professional standards of care.

PROCESS OF DIAGNOSING

The actual diagnosis of the client's problems involves the following:

1. Analyzing the data that were collected and sorted during the assessment phase
2. Identifying the client's actual and potential problems
3. Wording the identified problems in the correct format
4. Prioritizing the nursing diagnoses

Data analysis

In the assessment phase data were collected from a variety of sources and then sorted into clusters or categories given meaning by the system of sorting used. The nurse now needs to analyze or draw inferences from these clusters of data, using nursing knowledge and experience. This involves recognizing patterns or trends, comparing with normal healthful standards, and coming to a reasoned conclusion about the client's response to the illness or condition.

Example

Data cluster   Twenty-year-old female, first baby, wants to breast-feed; asking many questions about breast-feeding; has not attempted to breast-feed baby

Normal   Breast-feeding is a natural activity

Inference   Anxiety, knowledge deficit

Problem identification

The definition of a nursing diagnosis specifies concern for a client's actual or potential unhealthful responses to a condition or illness. It would thus not be appropriate to write a diagnosis for a one-time problem, such as a headache, since that is probably a coincidence rather than a response to an illness. Recurrent headaches, on the other hand, may justify writing a diagnosis, *if they are the client's response to an illness or condition.*

Generally, a nurse should write a diagnosis when a client is *actually* experiencing or will *potentially* experience a problem. *Actual* and *potential* describe the existing state of the client problem. By indicating the status of the problem the nurse also implies the type of nursing actions required for problem resolution or prevention.

Actual problems are those currently active; the client is experiencing the problem.

The data actually exist and have been identified as defining characteristics of the nursing diagnosis. Generally, the word "actual"
is not written: the diagnosis is presumed to
be an existing problem if the status is not
specified, as reflected in the following example.

Example

Existing defining characteristics   Dyspnea, tachy-
  pnea, shortness of breath, shallow respirations,
  nasal flaring, statements of worry, rapid and
  loud speech, muscular tension
Nursing diagnosis   Ineffective breathing pattern related to anxiety

It is worth noting that validating data must
exist for both parts of the nursing diagnosis:
the problem and the etiology. In the preceding example the cluster of symptoms indicating the problem was dyspnea, tachy-
pnea, shortness of breath, nasal flaring, and
shallow respirations. The etiology was validated by the symptoms of worry, rapid and
loud speech, and muscular tension. From
analysis of the assessed data, the nurse can
group symptoms and judge which cluster is
the unhealthful response to a condition (as
identified in the defining characteristics)
and which are the contributing factors (as

listed under possible etiologies). Whenever an actual problem diagnosis is written, the nurse needs to order and implement corrective actions to resolve the problem.

Potential problems are those states in which the contributing factors (etiology) exist, but the unhealthful response (problem) has not yet occurred. The client is at *high* risk for developing the problem. In this case the word "potential" is included in the nursing diagnosis statement, as shown in the following example.

Example

Existing defining characteristics Newly diagnosed diabetic client, states does not want "shots"; unable to state action of insulin or relationship to the disease process

Nursing diagnosis Potential for noncompliance with insulin treatment related to knowledge deficit of disease process and treatment

The purpose of writing a potential nursing diagnosis is to prevent the problem from actually occurring. By identifying a potential problem the nurse plans to forestall the development of an actual problem by alleviating the etiologic factors. In this case nursing interventions are preventive.

Format

Nursing diagnoses are the result of an educated analysis of assessed client data. After collecting the data the nurse sifts through the information, separates it into categories or areas of concern, examines it for contributing or associated factors, and finally establishes a diagnosis. The next step entails writing the statement in a professionally and legally acceptable style.

The properly written nursing diagnosis has two components: the problem and the etiology. These are connected by the phrase "related to" (r/t) or "associated with." Figure 2 illustrates both the relationship among the parts of the diagnostic statement and the format.

The problem, or title part, of the diagnostic statement is the identified unhealthful response of the client. It states what is wrong with the client from nursing's point of view. The list of nursing diagnoses, contained in Appendix B, is currently recognized by the North American Nursing Diagnosis Association (NANDA) as problems that nurses can diagnose and treat. The following reflect correct and incorrect diagnostic statements:

Problem ———⟶ related to → Etiology

Dysfunctional ——⟶ related to → Influencing or
  health pattern   associated factors

Potential for ——⟶ related to → Confusion
  injury

Fig. 2. *Relationship between the diagnostic statement and format.*

Incorrect problem statement	Tiredness
Correct problem statement	Sleep-pattern disturbance

The connecting phrase *related to* (r/t) establishes a relationship between the problem and the etiology. Although not implying a strict cause and effect relationship, the statement presents the etiology as an associated or contributing factor to the problem. It also enables the nurse to avoid legally or professionally inadvisable statements. The following provides examples of correct and incorrect establishment of the relationship between problem and etiology:

Incorrect relationship	Sleep-pattern disturbance *due to* . . .

Correct relationship   Sleep-pattern disturbance *r/t . . .*

The etiology part of the diagnostic statement contains individual client factors that are associated with, most likely causing, or contributing to the problem. The etiologic statement should not describe the symptoms of the problem; it should identify the factor(s) most strongly contributing to the client's problem. Because the etiology contributes to the problem, nursing interventions are focused on altering the etiology, which should in turn resolve the problem. NANDA has developed a list of the most frequently occurring etiologic factors for most of the accepted nursing diagnoses. The following are examples of incorrect and correct etiologies paired with diagnoses:

Incorrect etiology   Sleep-pattern disturbance r/t *inability to fall asleep*

Correct etiology   Sleep-pattern disturbance r/t *environmental change*

The following is an example of the perfectly acceptable practice of identifying more than one contributing factor when writing an etiology:

Alteration in nutrition, less than body requirements r/t nausea and stomatitis

Here the multiple etiology directs nursing interventions toward both of the contributing factors. Alleviating only the nausea, or the stomatitis, would not completely resolve the problem.

Sometimes the nurse finds it difficult to word an etiology concisely. Perhaps the etiology is complex or has a very specific complication. It is more important for the etiologic statement to be precise than concise. Since the purpose of the etiology is to direct the focus of nursing interventions, clarity and specificity take precedence over brevity. One way of dealing with the need to explain further is to add an explanation at the end of the etiology. This is usually done by using the phrase "secondary to," as in the following example:

Alteration in nutrition, less than body requirements r/t anorexia secondary to chemotherapy

"Secondary to" gives precise information about the nature of the anorexia and thus indicates more specific and efficient nursing care than if the etiology had been written simply as "anorexia." "Secondary to" indicates the specific origin of the etiology. Many times, however, it is not necessary or possible to include it, since the etiology itself is sufficiently specific, or the causative factor is unknown.

Rarely, the nurse writes a diagnostic statement and lists the etiology as "etiology unknown." This indicates that, although a problem exists, the nurse must continue to assess for contributing factors. In the meantime only general interventions directed at the signs and symptoms of the problem can be implemented.

PRIORITIZATION

After analyzing the assessment data the nurse identifies a number of client problems and decides how they should be listed on the care plan. In the clinical facility, nursing diagnoses are usually listed chronologically. When initiating the original care plan the nurse should prioritize the diagnoses and place the most pressing problems first. Thereafter, additional nursing diagnoses are simply added to the problem list. This system, in addition to changes in the client's status, eventually results in a problem list in which the priorities of client problems are out of order. When reviewing the problem list, despite the chronologic order, the nurse must identify which problems presently have the greatest priority.

When completing a care plan assignment, the student should enter the identified nursing diagnoses in descending order of priority. Since care plans are usually required only once for each client, the problems of ongoing identification and listing nursing diagnoses chronologically are bypassed.

A number of methods can be used to prioritize identified client problems. Nursing models, each based on a particular philosophy and viewpoint, have an intrinsic order of precedence that should be used to prioritize the client's problems. A common method of setting priorities follows the biopsychosocial approach and simply involves looking for the most life-threatening problems, followed by those that interfere with normal life functioning, and then those concerned with quality of life.

Abraham Maslow's hierarchy of needs is perhaps the most frequently used method of prioritizing nursing diagnoses. According to Maslow an intrinsic order exists in the immediacy of human needs, proceeding sequentially from the most basic biologic necessities to those of self-actualization. Whereas a person may have needs in each category at the same time, the most fundamental need has the greatest urgency. In most cases physiologic stability must be ensured before progress can be made in psychosocial areas. Lower-level needs always remain; however, when these needs are easily met, the needs-tension is reduced, and the person can then exert greater energy to meet higher-level needs.

Maslow lists the urgency of human needs in order of priority as follows:

Need	*Definition*
Physiologic	Biologic functions
Safety and security	Physical and emotional integrity from external threats
Love and belonging	Sense of interpersonal connectedness
Self-esteem	Positive view of self
Self-actualization	Personal growth and achievement and realization of potential; also spiritual needs

When the nurse formulates the original care plan, nursing diagnoses should be listed in order of priority. Therefore the nurse examines the problem portion of each diagnosis to see under which of Maslow's categories it belongs. They are then numbered in sequence, proceeding from the most basic physiologic problems. In this way the nurse can determine the priorities of nursing care. Usually the nurse must first ensure biologic functioning before advancing to psychosocial needs. An example of prioritizing follows.

Unprioritized nursing diagnoses
Self-care deficit r/t impaired mobility of left arm secondary to mastectomy
Alteration in nutrition, less than body requirements r/t nausea and vomiting
Potential for fluid and electrolyte imbalance r/t excessive vomiting
Body-image disturbance r/t perceived unattractiveness secondary to mastectomy
Potential for sexual dysfunction r/t feelings of undesirability
Potential for injury r/t sensory deficit in left hand
Spiritual distress r/t grieving over lost breast and diagnosis of metastatic cancer
Prioritized nursing diagnoses
Physiologic
Alteration in nutrition, less than body requirements r/t nausea and vomiting

Self-care deficit r/t impaired mobility of
left arm secondary to mastectomy

Potential for fluid and electrolyte imbalance r/t excessive vomiting

Safety and security

Potential for injury r/t sensory deficit in
left hand

Love and belonging

Potential for sexual dysfunction r/t feelings of undesirability

Self-esteem

Body-image disturbance r/t perceived unattractiveness secondary to mastectomy

Self-actualization

Spiritual distress r/t grieving over lost
breast and diagnosis of metastatic cancer

HELPFUL HINTS
Using a nursing diagnosis manual

Nursing diagnosis manuals, such as those
by Gordon and Carpenito, assist the nurse
in ensuring correct problem identification.
Accepted nursing diagnoses are listed, each
accompanied by its definition, possible etiologic factors, and expected signs and symptoms. When consulting a nursing diagnosis
manual the nurse should use the following
steps for writing a nursing diagnosis according to the NANDA format:

1. Check the definition of the nursing

diagnosis to see if that problem statement precisely describes what had been anticipated.

2. Check the listed defining characteristics against the client's signs and symptoms. The nursing diagnosis can be confirmed as accurate if several of the defining characteristics are present in the client data.

3. Examine the list of etiologic factors to see if the client presents one factor or more.

When the client problem matches the diagnosis definition, the data occur as listed under the defining characteristics and one etiologic factor or more are present, and the nurse can write the nursing diagnosis with confidence.

Example

Assessed client signs and symptoms

Right-sided weakness; unable to grasp with right hand or raise right arm; hair uncombed; teeth have food particles; medical diagnosis of cerebrovascular accident (CVA)

Nursing diagnosis category

Self-grooming deficit

Nursing diagnosis definition

Inability to dress or groom self

Defining characteristics

Impaired ability to put on or take off necessary clothing; inability to fasten clothing; inability to maintain appearance at satisfactory level; inability to provide adequate hygiene

Etiologic factors

Perceptual-cognitive impairment; activity intolerance; pain; neuromuscular impairment; musculoskeletal impairment

According to the assessed data the diagnosis definition matches the client problem. Several of the defining characteristics are found in the client's signs and symptoms, and the etiologic factor of neuromuscular impairment is present. Consequently, the nurse should write the nursing diagnosis as follows:

Self-grooming deficit r/t right-sided neuromuscular weakness secondary to cerebrovascular accident

Avoiding errors

Nursing diagnoses are easy to write if the nurse remembers that the problem portion of the diagnostic statement is concerned with the client's response to the illness or condition and that both the problem and etiology portions must be within the scope of nursing to diagnose and treat. The following suggestions should help the nurse prevent the most common errors in formulating nursing diagnoses:

1. Identify the client's response, not the medical diagnosis.
   a. *Incorrect nursing diagnosis*—Pain r/t myocardial infarction
   b. *Correct nursing diagnosis*—Pain r/t excessive physical exertion
2. Identify the problem created by the condition rather than the condition itself.
   a. *Incorrect nursing diagnosis*—Pain r/t surgery
   b. *Correct nursing diagnosis*—Activity intolerance r/t pain secondary to surgical incision
3. Identify the diagnostic category rather than the symptom.
   a. *Incorrect nursing diagnosis*—Cough r/t excessive mucus production
   b. *Correct nursing diagnosis*—Altered breathing pattern r/t excessive mucus production
4. Identify a treatable etiology rather than a clinical sign.
   a. *Incorrect nursing diagnosis*—Altered respiratory function r/t abnormal arterial blood gases (ABGs)
   b. *Correct nursing diagnosis*—Altered respiratory function r/t ventilation-perfusion imbalance

5. Identify the problem brought about by the diagnostic study rather than the study itself.
   a. *Incorrect nursing diagnosis*—Anxiety r/t cardiac catheterization
   b. *Correct nursing diagnosis*—Anxiety r/t lack of knowledge about cardiac catheterization
6. Identify the client response to the equipment rather than the equipment itself.
   a. *Incorrect nursing diagnosis*—Anxiety r/t cardiac monitor
   b. *Correct nursing diagnosis*—Sleep-pattern disturbance r/t anxiety about need for cardiac monitoring
7. Identify the client's problems rather than those of the nurse.
   a. *Incorrect nursing diagnosis*—Potential IV problems r/t poor vascular access
   b. *Correct nursing diagnosis*—Potential for infection r/t presence of invasive lines
8. Identify the client problem rather than the nursing intervention.
   a. *Incorrect nursing diagnosis*—Potential fluid volume excess r/t need to limit fluids
   b. *Correct nursing diagnosis*—Potential fluid volume excess r/t noncompliance with fluid restrictions
9. Identify the client problem rather than the client goal.

   a. *Incorrect nursing diagnosis*—Noncompliance r/t need to quit smoking
   b. *Correct nursing diagnosis*—Alteration in health maintenance r/t knowledge deficit about dangers of smoking.
10. Make professional judgments rather than prejudicial ones.
   a. *Incorrect nursing diagnosis*—Refusal to comply with treatment r/t anger
   b. *Correct nursing diagnosis*—Noncompliance with treatment r/t anxiety secondary to knowledge deficit of disease process and treatment
11. Identify associated factors; avoid legally inadvisable statements.
   a. *Incorrect nursing diagnosis*—Recurrent angina r/t insufficient medication
   b. *Correct nursing diagnosis*—Recurrent chest pain r/t noncompliance with medications secondary to knowledge decifit of information resources
12. Identify both the *problem* and the *etiology*. Be careful to avoid a circular statement.
   a. *Incorrect nursing diagnosis*—Alteration in comfort r/t pain
   b. *Correct nursing diagnosis*—Altered breathing pattern r/t pain

Identifying the real problem

   Occasionally the nurse, when formulating the diagnostic statement, is at an impasse. Although believeing that the problem has been diagnosed, the nurse identifies an etiology that breaks one of the preceding rules. Surgical clients frequently present this dilemma. The nurse is aware of the client's postoperative pain and is tempted to write the following incorrect diagnosis:

Alteration in comfort: pain r/t incision

Is this the real problem? The pain is an outcome of the treatment of the illness, as is the incision. The trick is to analyze the client's response further to find the unhealthful behavior. How is the client reacting to the incisional pain? Is the client refusing to cough and deep breathe or reluctant to ambulate? These are actual *responses* to the condition of having a painful incision.

To resolve this situation the nurse should turn the diagnostic statement around, that is, describe the supposed problem as the etiology. Very often the real problem (unhealthful response) becomes immediately evident. Suddenly the nursing diagnosis makes sense *and* can be legally diagnosed and treated by the nurse. The nurse now correctly writes the following:

Noncompliance with postoperative regimen r/t incisional pain

It is also perfectly acceptable to use a nursing diagnosis (as defined by NANDA) as an etiology, as in the following example:

Potential for altered respiratory function r/t noncompliance with postoperative regimen.

SUMMARY

A nursing diagnosis is a statement in which the nurse identifies the client's response to an unhealthful condition based on an analysis of the collected data. The purpose of making a nursing diagnosis is to identify client problems to provide a basis for formulating a treatment plan. Both the diagnosis and the treatment plan must be educationally and legally within the domain of nursing practice.

There are four criteria for writing a nursing diagnosis accurately: the identified problem must be the client's response to an illness or unhealthful situation; the problem must be of a level that requires professional knowledge and analysis; it must be within the scope of nursing practice to identify; and it must be within the legal domain of nursing practice to treat.

The process of diagnosing client problems involves analyzing the data base, identifying the client's actual and potential problems, wording the problem statement accurately, and prioritizing the identified problems to organize nursing care.

The diagnostic statement has two parts: problem and etiology. The problem portion is the client's dysfunctional health pattern. The etiology states the factor or condition that is associated with or contributing to the problem. These two parts are connected by the phrase "related to."

Writing nursing diagnoses takes practice. When beginning the nurse needs to follow the rules, use the standardized statements formulated by NANDA, and keep in mind that it is the client's response to the illness or condition that is being looked for to identify a problem that is within the scope of nursing to treat. The etiology must be precise and descriptive and cannot contain legal or professional misstatements.

Properly written nursing diagnoses benefit both the client and the nurse. They center attention and care on the client's problems in an organized manner, thereby meeting the client's needs more effectively.

Nurses benefit by using standardized nursing diagnoses, since each nurse understands the client's identified problems in the same way, facilitating communication and organization of care delivery.

BIBLIOGRAPHY

Anderson JE and Briggs LL: Nursing diagnosis: a study of quality and supportive evidence, Image 20:141, 1988.

Atkinson LD and Murray ME: Understanding the nursing process, ed 3, New York, 1986, Macmillan Publishing Co.

Carpenito LJ: Handbook of nursing diagnoses, ed 2, Philadelphia, 1987, JB Lippincott Co.

Carpenito LJ: Nursing diagnosis: application to clinical practice, ed 2, Philadelphia, 1987, JB Lippincott Co.

Fraher JE: Nursing diagnoses and care plans in critical care, Crit Care Nurs 3:94, 1983.

Gordon M: Manual of nursing diagnosis, New York, 1985, McGraw-Hill, Inc.

Kim MJ and Moritz DA, editors: Classification of nursing diagnoses, New York, 1982, McGraw-Hill, Inc.

North American Nursing Diagnosis Association: NANDA approved nursing diagnosis categories, Nursing Diagnosis Newsletter 15:1, 1988.

Tartaglia MJ: Nursing diagnosis: keystone of your care plan, Nursing85 34:36, 1985.

NURSING CARE PLAN

Discharge Goal:

ASSESSMENT	NURSING DIAGNOSIS
Subjective data 　Interview	Problem related to 　etiology
Objective data 　Physical examination 　Health record 　Observation of be- 　　havior 　Other sources	Problem—Client re- 　sponse to illness or 　medical treatment
Data organization	Etiology—Causative or 　associated factor(s) 　within scope of nurs- 　ing practice

EXPECTED OUTCOMES   INTERVENTIONS   EVALUATION

4

Planning

- **Setting goals**
- **Selecting interventions**
- **Documentation**

The planning phase of the nursing process initiates nursing management of client care. Assessment and diagnosis required gathering facts and identifying client problems. Actions have not yet been taken to change the client's condition. In the planning step the nurse prepares to intervene on the client's behalf, formulating specific goals and interventions to meet the client's needs.

The client care plan is written during the planning step. Since it is a written document and part of the client's legal medical record, the care plan must be individualized to the client for whom it is written. The two previous steps of the nursing process (assessment and diagnosis) are the means by which this individualization of the care plan occurs. The components of the planning step are developing expected outcomes, selecting intervention strategies, and communicating the care plan.

EXPECTED OUTCOMES

Expected outcomes, or goals, are client behaviors or responses that the nurse anticipates occurring as a result of nursing interventions. They are specific statements indicating how the nurse expects resolution of the client's problem. After the nurse has assessed and diagnosed the client's problems, goal statements are formulated for the overall client outcome and for each identified client problem. The nurse uses these statements to evaluate the client's condition and behavior after the implementation phase.

The terminology and procedure for writing goal statements vary in nursing literature. Although many terms are used, only two major approaches for writing expected outcomes exist.

One approach involves a two-step process: a general goal statement is given, and specific outcome criteria are written indicating behaviors by which the nurse evaluates whether the goal was met.

The second method, which this text favors, simplifies the process by naming specific expected behaviors in the goal statement. This approach is consistent with documentation requirements in most facilities, which opt for the fewest number of statements whenever possible. Furthermore, the one-step method reduces the possibility of a subjective nursing interpretation of the general goal statement replacing an objective nursing evaluation of the outcome criteria. In the one-step method the evaluation criteria are contained in the goal statement. The nurse specifies in a single statement the exact behaviors or responses that are expected to occur as a result of planned nursing interventions.

How to write a goal statement

The format for writing a goal is specified by the criteria, which are the rules to follow when writing a goal, the "how-to" instructions. They eliminate vagueness and subjective judgments during evaluation. Because they are concerned with responses that the nurse does not see yet but hopes to see later, goal statements are always written in the future tense. When correctly formulated the goal statement specifies *who* will do *what, how, when,* and to *what degree.* The following criteria should be considered when writing a goal:

1. Client centered
2. Singular
3. Observable
4. Measurable
5. Time limited
6. Mutual
7. Realistic

Client centered

Since the entire thrust of the care plan is toward correcting the client's problems, it naturally follows that the expected outcomes are also focused on the client. The goal statement should reflect those client behaviors or responses that the nurse expects to occur as a result of nursing interventions.

When writing a goal the nurse should be careful when specifying what is expected from the client. The most common errors in writing expected outcomes occur when the focus is shifted to the nurse. This results in a *nursing* goal. The following provides examples of incorrect and correct formulations of an expected outcome:

Incorrect   The client will be offered 120 cc H_2O qh.

Correct   The client will drink 120 cc H_2O qh.

The difference between the correct and incorrect version is in *who* will perform the action. Although a goal statement may begin with the phrase "the client will," the nurse's focus may not be on the client. In the incorrect goal statement the client is the passive object of the action. When correctly written the goal statement specifies that the client will be expected to actively do something.

Singular

Each goal statement should specify one, and only one, expected outcome. If two or more behavior changes are anticipated, the nurse should write them as separate goals. This prevents confusion and subjective judgments during the evaluation phase. The following examples illustrate this criterion:

Incorrect   The client will eat 100% of diet and lose no weight by discharge.

Correct   The client will eat 100% of diet by 6/20. The client will maintain weight of 120 lbs. until discharge.

The incorrect goal statement identifies two responses for the nurse to evaluate. Should the client eat only a portion of the diet but not lose any weight, the nurse will have difficulty determining if the goal was met. A subjective judgment would have to be made. By dividing the expected behaviors into separate goal statements the nurse eliminates the decisional element in evaluating the goal. The nurse simply observes if the behavior or response occurred.

The number of goals needed depends on the manner in which the nursing diagnosis is written. The nurse should write as many expected outcomes as necessary to resolve the problem. It is more important that each goal have only one behavior than to have only one or two goals.

Observable

The desired result, as stated in the goal, must be perceivable. If the nurse has no way to identify if the response occurred, it is impossible to evaluate whether the goal was achieved. This may seem obvious: no one would write a goal for something they could not see or evaluate. However, the problem occurs when dealing with two major areas: the client's knowledge and emotions.

If a nursing diagnosis was written regarding a knowledge deficit, the nurse may be tempted to write the following:

Incorrect   The client will understand how to change the colostomy appliance in 1 wk.

Correct   The client will demonstrate understanding by correctly changing the colostomy appliance within 1 wk.

Knowing and understanding are not visible to the observer. What is visible is the behavior illustrating the acquired knowledge or understanding. Asking clients about their knowledge or understanding does not result in objective data; clients must actually demonstrate understanding by using the acquired knowledge. The signs (lack of knowledgeable behaviors) that led the nurse to make the nursing diagnosis can be used to formulate the goal statements.

A similar difficulty arises when dealing with a client's emotions. Should a nursing diagnosis be written about the client's anxiety, for example, the nurse may want to state the following:

Incorrect	Preoperative anxiety will be relieved by the morning of surgery.
Correct	On the morning of surgery the client will demonstrate that anxiety has been relieved by stating all questions have been answered.

Nobody can actually verify another's emotions, thoughts, or abilities. The nurse must rely on the client's statement about personal feelings or compare present behavior with the previous behavior that led to the nursing diagnosis. The goal is then written to specify a behavior or statement that can be objectively observed as occurring. Abilities are verified only by actual client demonstration. Statements such as "will be able to" should be avoided. Only what the client *does*, not what the client is able to do, is observable, as illustrated in the following example:

Incorrect	The client will be able to plan 1500 calorie American Diabetes Association (ADA) menu in 1 wk.
Correct	The client will plan 1 day's menu for 1500 calorie ADA diet by 1 wk.

Measurable

Expected outcomes are written to give the nurse a standard against which the client's response to interventions can be measured. When the goal is vague or unmeasurable, the nurse can evaluate only the client's response in a subjective manner. Words such as "normal" and "sufficient" mean different things to different people, and each person would evaluate differently a goal written in such an ambiguous manner.

When a goal is measurably stated, the nurse can quantify, or measure, the desired response objectively. The behavior can be judged as happening or not happening; the amount or frequency can be counted, measured, or weighed. Since many kinds of

things require measurement, several examples of nonmeasurable and measurable
goals follow.

Example 1

Incorrect   The client will ambulate more qd.
Correct   The client will ambulate 20 ft. in the
hallway by 8/3. The client will ambulate
10 ft. further in the hallway qd beginning
8/4; *or*, The client will ambulate at least tid by
8/4.

In the incorrect example the word "more"
is ambiguous. Increased ambulation is desired, but it is not known whether "more"
means an increase in frequency or distance.
Correct examples given for both measures
identify exactly how the increase is to be
measured.

Example 2

Incorrect   The client will have an acceptable
blood pressure by 2/11.
Correct   The client's systolic blood pressure
will be < 160 by 2/11.

Here the vague word is "acceptable." The
nurse who wrote the goal may have a clear
idea what blood pressure is acceptable
for this client, but that measurement

was not communicated. Numbers should be provided so the evaluating nurse will have a precise yardstick with which to measure.

Example 3

Incorrect   The client will accurately describe a low-salt diet in 3 days.

Correct   The client will identify at least three foods recommended on a low-salt diet in 3 days. The client will name at least three foods to be avoided on a low-salt diet in 3 days.

"Accurately" is the ambiguous term in this example, since accuracy has variable degrees. Exactly what and how much information the client should demonstrate need to be specifically stated.

Example 4

Incorrect   The client will have a decrease in pain by 6/13.

Correct   The client will state she has less pain by 6/13; *or,* The client will demonstrate a decrease in pain by requesting pain medication less than qid by 6/13.

The incorrect goal here does not inform the nurse what measure to use during evaluation. The first correct example gives a "yes-

or-no" method of evaluation; the client either expresses or does not express a decrease in pain. The second correct example
gives an evaluation tool (pain medication re-
quests) and a measure (less than four times
a day). The kind of measurement and, when
necessary, the amount to be measured are
essential items in the goal statement.

Each of the above examples illustrates a
different type of measurement. No matter
what behavior or response is desired, objective evaluation is made possible by quanti-
fying the goal statement. A measurable goal
enables the nurse to evaluate whether the
goal was met at all, was partially met, or was
completely met. It eliminates guesswork and
ensures consistency of treatment and evaluation.

Time limited

Every goal statement should specify a
time frame, which indicates when the expected response should occur or when the
nurse should examine for progress in the
area. Without a time reference the nurse has
no standard to judge whether progress is
being made at a reasonable rate.

Example 1

Incorrect The client will breast-feed her baby.
Correct The client will breast-feed her baby q3h by 10/8.

The incorrect example specifies a behavior but not the frequency or terminal date by which it should occur. Depending on the situation the frequency of the expected behavior may be omitted in the goal statement, as illustrated in the following example. However, the terminal date for evaluation must always be included.

Example 2

Incorrect The client will state tid a determination to cease smoking by 1/17.
Correct The client will state by 1/17 a determination to cease smoking; *or,* The client will state by 1/17 a determination to quit smoking by 2/1.

Some behaviors or responses do not require repetition. The incorrect example above has two errors. First, the client does not need to repeat three times a day a willingness to stop smoking. The second error is one of ambiguity. Does the statement mean that the client will cease smoking by 1/17 or that a statement of intent will be made by that date? The evaluation date should be placed anywhere in the goal statement that makes intent clear. The second correct goal specifies both the expected date of the client statement and the date of the anticipated cessation of smoking.

The time limit in the goal assists the nurse in keeping priorities in perspective. Often goals are set in stepwise fashion, with one behavior expected to occur before the next. This is easily accomplished by placing sequential dates in the goal statements.

When the date of evaluation, as specified in the goal, arrives, the nurse assesses for completion of the desired behavior or response. If the nurse judges that the goal is still appropriate but not completely met, a new evaluation date may be set.

Mutual

The entire care plan has the greatest chance of a successful outcome if it is planned by the nurse and the client together. Mutual goal setting ensures that both the client and nurse agree on what needs to be accomplished and in what

amount of time. By establishing the expected outcomes together the nurse involves the client as an active participant in
care and thereby increases client cooperation.

When establishing goals the nurse is in
danger of imposing personal values on the
client. The nurse's role here is to present
the client with the available options, to give
information and advice based on nursing
knowledge and experience, and finally to
work collaboratively with the client to establish mutually agreeable goals. Both the
client and the nurse will know what to expect. Conflict and frustration will be prevented. Mutual respect increases as the
nurse and client work together. This results
in attainable goals because the client is mo-
tivated to work for those things she or he
values and has helped to plan.

Realistic

No matter how perfectly a goal is stated,
if it is not attainable, it is not a good goal.
Although some desired outcomes may be
ideal, they may not be realistic for a particular client. Some ideal outcomes may not be

possible for a particular client for two general reasons: poor prognosis and conflicting values.

In the first case a client's physical condition may be such that striving for complete recovery is unrealistic. Chronic diseases, such as chronic obstructive pulmonary disease and rheumatoid arthritis, are examples of permanently compromising physical conditions. Realistic outcomes in situations such as these should focus on helping the client maintain whatever capabilities remain and adjust to any new losses.

When values conflict, the nurse must eventually defer to the client's wishes. It is simply unrealistic to work for something the client does not want. As discussed earlier, goal setting should be a mutual process. It may be possible, for instance, for an elderly client with a hip fracture to walk again; however, if the client is unwilling to expend the effort and is content to be wheelchair bound, it would be better for the nurse to concentrate on assisting the client to live capably in a wheelchair. The nurse, in a case such as this, has the obligation to help the client understand that ambulation is possible. In the end, however, a decision based on knowledge of the alternatives is the right of the client. The realistic nurse accepts the decision and works to maximize the client's potential at whatever level the client decides.

When to write a goal statement

The three types of expected outcomes in a care plan are (1) discharge goals, (2) long-term goals, and (3) short-term goals. Although each of these goals has a different purpose, they are written in the same format, using the criteria discussed in the previous section, "How to Write a Goal Statement."

Figure 3 illustrates the relationship of the parts of the care plan to the different kinds of goals.

Discharge goals

A discharge goal is the overall expected client outcome following admission for health care, that is, the desired end result of the entire care plan. A care plan usually includes several problems, each of which has its own set of goals. The discharge goal is a

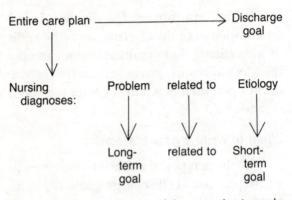

Fig. 3. Relationship of parts of the care plan to goals.

summary of these goals. It states in what condition and to where the patient is expected to be discharged.

Most facilities have standardized care plan forms. The space for the discharge goal is usually at the top of the page, and it may be labeled "Discharge Planning" or "Overall Long-Term Goal." In some facilities a blank space is provided for the nurse to write the discharge goal. In others, general discharge goals are preprinted and the nurse simply indicates which goal is appropriate for the client.

The following are three general types of discharge outcomes:

1. Discharge without limitations/life-style changes to home/extended care facility (ECF)/other
2. Discharge with limitations/life-style changes to home/ECF/other
3. Death with comfort and dignity

If the discharge goals are preprinted on the facility's care plan form, the nurse selects the one appropriate for the particular client. Place of discharge or limitations and life-style changes can be specified as needed. If a blank space is given for discharge planning on the care plan form, the goal is stated in the standard format, using one of the previously listed alternatives.

It is understood when writing expected outcomes that the client is expected to perform the activity and achieve the stated result. Therefore the phrase "the client" may be omitted from the goal statement.

The purpose of the discharge goal is to coordinate care so that the entire health-care team works with the same overall purpose in mind. It helps to keep things in perspective while working on the individual problems.

Long-term goals

As indicated in Figure 3 long-term goals (LTGs) are concerned with the problem portion of the nursing diagnosis. Each nursing diagnosis in the care plan has its own LTG. The LTG is usually the reverse of the problem; it states elements indicating problem resolution.

The problem portion of the nursing diagnosis, as described in Chapter 3, states the client's unhealthful response to the illness or condition. The nurse eventually wants to change this unhealthful response. The LTG identifies the anticipated outcome for the particular unhealthful response.

Example

Nursing diagnosis   Alteration in skin integrity: rash r/t use of irritating detergents

LTG   Within 1 wk. skin will be free of rash

The time element of the LTG depends on the nature of the problem, the etiology, and the overall condition of the client. Some problems are readily resolved because the etiology is uncomplicated and the client's condition is generally good. Other problems take longer to resolve; either the etiology is complicated or the client's condition is poor and improvement is slow.

The setting in which the client is treated also affects the time element of goals. In general the LTG is shorter in duration in the special care areas of a hospital. The client in labor and delivery or in the emergency department will not be there for a week, yet nursing diagnoses are written. LTGs in these settings are set in terms of hours rather than days or weeks.

Example

Nursing diagnosis   Alteration in comfort: pain r/t vaginal stretching during labor
LTG   Will state pain is significantly relieved within 1h

Clients in rehabilitation facilities and outpatient clinics usually have continuing or chronic conditions that require extended treatment; therefore LTGs are frequently set in terms of months.

Example

Nursing diagnosis   Impaired mobility: ambulation r/t left-sided weakness secondary to CVA
LTG   Will walk 50 ft. unaided within 4 mos

Nursing diagnoses are written as actual or potential problems. When an actual nursing diagnosis is identified, the LTG is focused on reversing the problem. Potential problems are those that have not yet occurred. For these diagnoses the LTG is concerned with preventing occurrence or maintaining the client's status to prevent the problem.

Example

Nursing diagnosis   Potential for injury: falling r/t vertigo

LTG   Will not fall or injure self throughout the hospital stay

Nursing diagnosis   Potential alteration in nutrition, more than body requirements r/t food intake–energy expenditure imbalance

LTG   Will maintain weight between 120 and 125 lbs. throughout treatment

When the LTG is met, the problem no longer actively exists. The particular nursing diagnosis is then discontinued on the care plan.

Short-term goals

Figure 3 shows that short-term goals (STGs) focus on the etiology of the nursing diagnosis. More than one STG is usually indicated for each diagnostic statement.

As discussed in Chapter 3, the etiology portion of the nursing diagnosis identifies the factor(s) associated with or causing the problem. If the cause is removed, the problem will cease to exist. STGs are concerned with altering or removing the causative factor(s) and thereby resolving the problem. STGs are the "working" part of the care plan.

A word of caution is necessary: for the actual resolution of the problem the etiology must be correctly identified. If the etiology is incorrect, no matter how successful the client is in meeting the STGs, the problem will not be resolved. It is therefore important when writing STGs to keep in mind the relationship between the problem and the etiology.

LTGs are singular statements indicating problem resolution. STGs, on the other hand, are small step-by-step objectives that cumulatively lead to the elimination of the etiology and thus the problem. A series of sequential STGs is indicated for most etiologies. Each STG should successively come closer to resolving the cause of the problem.

Multiple STGs are formulated because very few things can be solved by a single action. Almost every task, from tying shoelaces to writing a care plan, requires multiple abilities and activities. Step-by-step STGs give the nurse practical guidance in planning interventions. If the STG is too global, the nurse will not have specific guidelines for what must be accomplished.

Example

Nursing diagnosis　　Alteration in health maintenance r/t lack of knowledge about diabetic care

Incorrect STG　　Client will accurately describe diabetic care in 1 wk.

Correct STGs
1. By the end of the first teaching session, client will explain the relationship between diet, exercise, and insulin.
2. By the end of the second teaching session, client will test blood for glucose using a glucometer.
3. By the end of the third teaching session, client will inject self with insulin.
4. By the end of the fourth teaching session, client will describe the techniques for foot care.
5. By the end of the fifth teaching session, client will plan one meal using the diabetic food exchange list.

6. Within 1 wk., client will state future use of all the identified techniques of diabetic care.

The number of STGs necessary depends on the etiology. The more precise the etiology and the fewer elements it contains, the fewer STGs will be needed.

Example

Nursing diagnosis   Alteration in health maintenance r/t lack of knowledge about rotating insulin injection sites

STGs

1. After the first teaching session, client will state two reasons for rotating insulin injection sites.
2. By the end of the second teaching session, client will identify five body parts where insulin may be injected.
3. By the end of the second teaching session, client will state intention to rotate injection sites using at least three body parts.

When writing STGs the nurse examines the etiology for its component parts in relation to the LTG. Upon breaking down these parts the nurse places them in an order reflecting when the client is to sequentially achieve all goals. The nurse knows that the STGs are sufficient when they not only resolve the etiology but also make the connection with the problem. STGs are written sequentially and subsequently assigned time frames. It is acceptable for STGs to be accomplished out of order, as long as the nurse reviews and verifies that the client has all the necessary abilities to maintain the newly acquired skills successfully.

INTERVENTION SELECTION

Once the expected outcomes are established, the process of selecting appropriate interventions begins. Choosing suitable nursing strategies is an educated decision-making process. The nurse judges which specific interventions will most successfully meet the goals. This judgment is based on the client's needs and abilities identified in the assessment and diagnostic phases and on the nurse's knowledge and experience of what is needed to meet the goals.

Selecting interventions is a deliberate process whereby appropriate strategies are chosen to achieve the STGs. As stated earlier the STGs are the operative focus of the care plan. All interventions are directed toward meeting the STGs, which in turn should re-

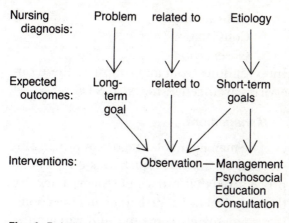

Fig. 4. *Relationship of interventions to expected outcomes.*

solve the problem. Each STG has its own set of interventions. Figure 4 illustrates the relationship of interventions to the established expected outcomes. It also indicates the types of interventions that make up the scope of nursing practice.

Types of interventions

The following are five types of nursing interventions, as indicated in Figure 4:

1. Management
2. Psychosocial

3. Education
4. Consultation
5. Observation

Interventions from all or most of these categories are needed for each STG.

Management

The management category of nursing interventions includes all hands-on physical procedures that nurses perform. They are the technical tasks, such as giving injections, that immediately come to mind when nursing practice is mentioned. This type of intervention is almost universally included when resolving the etiology. The only instances when management interventions may be excluded are when the etiology of the nursing diagnosis concerns knowledge deficit or psychosocial factors.

Nursing management can be independent, interdependent, or dependent. The differences reside in the source of authority for the action, as seen in the following examples of nursing procedures.

Independent	Active and passive range of motion (ROM) to all unaffected joints each shift

Interdependent	Nasopharyngeal suction-ing as required
Dependent	Medicate with Valium 10 mg po q6h

Psychosocial

Psychosocial nursing interventions have a supportive character and are concerned with the client's emotions and personal relationships. However, they are not the nursing substitute for psychologic or psychiatric counseling; rather, they are the professional awareness of and assistance to the client in recognizing and dealing with nonphysical responses to the illness and treatment. Psychosocial interventions help the client reestablish or maintain emotional equilibrium.

By their very nature psychosocial interventions are independent nursing activities. The nurse has been educated to identify, support, and promote healthy coping behaviors. This aspect of nursing practice is almost never medically ordered outside of psychiatric practice; it is assumed that it will be implemented as needed.

Psychosocial interventions should be part of the nursing orders for each STG. No matter what is being accomplished the client's feelings and commitment to the goal must be considered. The following examples of psychosocial interventions concern a patient's awareness of a problem, her fears about it, and how it affects her relationship with a significant other.

Awareness	Discuss with client the significance of her inability to bear children after the hysterectomy.
Fears	Provide uninterrupted time for client to express worries about undergoing major surgery.
Relationships	Provide opportunity and encourage client and significant other to talk about their feelings about adopting children in the future.

Education

The ANA's Standards of Nursing Practice (1976) and most states' nurse practice acts identify patient education as a legal professional nursing responsibility. Unless the client receives some form of health teaching, nursing care for that client is not considered adequate. The purpose of client education is to give the client sufficient knowledge and skills to increase participation in health care. This participation should extend from informed decision making to knowledge of complete self-care.

Health teaching can prevent, promote, maintain, modify, or increase health-related behaviors. It is a necessary concurrent intervention with management. Whenever something is done for a client, the information about what is being done and any related health behaviors should be taught. Failure to include this kind of health teaching leaves the client in a helpless and dependent position.

Client education includes formal and informal teaching. Formal teaching is the planned, organized presentation of health-care information, for example, preoperative instructions and prenatal classes. Informal teaching is the furnishing of information about health status or the spontaneous answering of a client's questions about health-care matters. Both approaches should be included in every care plan.

In most circumstances client education is an independent nursing function. It is expected to occur when appropriate as a normal part of nursing care delivery. Sometimes, however, the physician specifically orders a certain type or program of client teaching. This formal teaching, authorized by a medical order, is a dependent nursing activity. Also, when ancillary departments are involved during the course of care, the nurse reinforces information and instructions from the other disciplines. This teaching has an interdependent nature. The following gives examples of independent, dependent, and interdependent teaching.

Example

Independent   Instruct client to hold nitroglycerin (NTG) tablet under the tongue and not to chew or swallow it.

Dependent   Remind client to use incentive spirometer qh while awake, as directed by respiratory therapist.

Interdependent   Implement step 1 of cardiac rehabilitation program (standardized teaching plan) on 5/12.

Consultation

Consultation has two components: conferring and referring. The nurse confers with other health-care professionals about some aspect of the client's care. This kind of consultation is intended to enhance the nurse's expertise in caring for the client. The nurse also refers the client to other health-care professionals or another agency. Referrals give the client first-hand contact with an expert in the field. The expert can work intensively with the client on an individual basis. This kind of help is often extended beyond the time of the client's discharge from the nurse's care.

For a variety of reasons sometimes the expert with whom the nurse confers is the client's family or significant other. The significant other may have information or an insight that helps the nurse provide effective care. Very often the nurse needs to collaborate with the family or caretaker to ensure adequate preparation, equipment, and skills for assuming care of the client after discharge.

Consultation may be either an independent or dependent nursing function, depending on the nature of the consultation and the particular facility's policy. Because some third-party payment policies require a physician's order for consultation with professional services, the nurse may need to request an order for a consultation when it becomes necessary. Independent and dependent consultative nursing orders may be written as follows:

Independent	Consult with occupational therapy for projects that the client can do in bed to increase manual dexterity; *or,* confer with client's spouse about arranging client's bed on first floor so that client will not have to climb stairs.
Dependent	Request order from physician for referral to Reach for Recovery before discharge; *or,* Request dietitian to teach client and spouse about low-fat, low-salt diet before discharge, per physician request.

Observation

Observations, as depicted in Figure 4, are the only type of intervention that is not concentrated solely on the STGs. As indicated in Chapter 2 assessment is an ongoing, continuous activity throughout the nursing process. In the planning stage key indicators of the problem, the etiology, each short-term goal, and the client's response to each intervention are marked for continuous observation. The observation of all these factors is the connecting element. Management, psychosocial, education, and consultation interventions are related to the STG. Observation interventions keep the STGs in the perspective of the LTG. Continuous interactive observation makes it possible for the nurse to evaluate if the etiology has been alleviated and the problem resolved. The entire process is tied together by continuous monitoring of all aspects.

Another unique characteristic of observation as an intervention is its seeming lack of benefit to the client. Other interventions actively intermediate on the client's behalf. Observations actually do nothing for the client in concrete terms. Merely observing the client and responses changes nothing, yet observations are a critical part of planning effective implementation. By accurately pinpointing all the behaviors and responses requiring continuous monitoring, the nurse makes objective evaluation and pertinent readjustment possible.

Ongoing assessment is generally an independent nursing function. In most cases it is the nurse's responsibility to monitor the client's status and to report any untoward signs. After a bronchoscopy, for example, the nurse must monitor for return of the gag reflex. Before the procedure, in planning postprocedural care, the nurse writes the following:

Check for gag reflex and monitor q30min for return after bronchoscopy.

Although interdependent observations are nursing responsibilities, they also form the basis for medical treatment or require a medical order to treat if the assessment finds an abnormal response. As an example, interdependent observations are encountered when caring for the diabetic client. Because diabetes mellitus is a dysfunction in glucose metabolism, the nurse is automatically responsible for monitoring the client's blood glucose. If abnormally high blood glucose is present, the nurse needs a medical order to treat the condition. This is truly collaborative practice. The nurse then writes the following in the care plan:

Monitor blood glucose q4h; report results < 80 mg/dl or > 120 mg/dl to physician.

Critical care units are the areas where dependent observations are most commonly ordered. Frequently, standing orders are in effect, giving the nurse authority to act when certain abnormal conditions are present. These standardized procedures are preplanned medical orders created to meet critical or emergency situations. None of these interventions can be undertaken on the nurse's own authority; even instituting the assessments requires a physician's order, for example:

Hemodynamic monitoring qh; report results not within normal parameters to physician.

How to select interventions

Following familiarity with the types of interventions encompassing nursing practice, the nurse's next task is to decide which interventions will best resolve the client's problems. The solution has two facets. First, the types of intervention chosen depend on the difficulty or complexity of the problem. With these considerations in mind, the method of selecting interventions is then the same no matter what kind of problem it is. Next, by keeping the intensity of the client problem in mind the nurse has a clearer idea of how vigorous the interventions need to be and what types of interventions are best suited to problem resolution.

Level of problem

There are two types of nursing diagnoses, as discussed in Chapter 3: actual and potential. Each type indicates a different level of client problem and requires a different nursing approach.

Actual problems are those that the client is currently experiencing. These problems need active and aggressive management. The focus is on removing problematic behaviors and conditions and replacing them with healthful ones. All five categories of nursing interventions are generally required for actual problems.

Potential problems are those that have not yet occurred but almost certainly will if no corrective action is taken. Preventive nursing strategies are necessary. The nurse's intent must be to forestall the problem, that is, to interrupt the chain of events that will result in an actual problem if action is not taken. Again, all five intervention types may be required, but the emphasis is usually on education and observation.

Methods for intervention selection

The nurse uses three basic methods to generate all possible alternatives and then to finally select those interventions most suitable for the client. These methods include thinking of alternative interventions, researching textbooks and standardized care plans, and collaborating with other members of the health-care team and the client.

Thinking should be the nurse's first action when planning interventions. The nurse should reflect on what things need to be accomplished to meet this goal. Reflecting, remembering, devising, and brainstorming are all legitimate means of generating as many interventions as possible to meet the goal. The nurse uses the five types of interventions as guidelines to verify that the list is as complete as possible.

Researching textbooks, manuals, and standardized care plans should follow. Since these resources address the usual problems and solutions for given conditions, they are written in general terms and do not apply specifically to the client. However, these sources are valuable for comparing ideas and checking if anything important has been overlooked; these can then be added to the list of potential interventions.

The nurse should now have more interventions than necessary. Some interventions will be discarded as inappropriate, and others will be modified to adapt to the client's needs and abilities. The nurse fine-tunes the list of possible interventions, narrowing it down to those suitable for the client.

Collaborating completes the process of tailoring the interventions specifically to the client. The nurse collaborates with knowledgeable members of the health-care team and the client. Knowledgeable members of the health-care team are those who know and have cared for the client or who have expertise in the problem. Their advice and suggestions are important, and the nurse should consider their responses. Because each health-care team member has a role in the client's care, all interventions planned by the nurse must be congruent with those of the rest of the team.

The client provides the final information needed to select interventions most suitable for and acceptable to the client. Planned interventions contrary to a client's values or belief system will not be accepted. It is necessary to uncover what the client hopes and expects to achieve. Including the client's personal aims in the care plan ensures compliance during the implementation phase.

COMMUNICATION

Now that expected outcomes have been established and interventions selected, it is time to communicate the care plan to the client and to the health-care team. The care plan is both verbally communicated and written in the client's medical record. Effective communication makes the care plan work.

The client

After formulating the care plan the nurse should review it with the client. The client has the right and need to understand the focus of care and what is expected. This review affords one more opportunity to make sure that the client and nurse are in agreement. Mutual care planning increases trust between nurse and client and facilitates implementation.

Reviewing the care plan with the client does not mean reading the document verbatim. The nurse should verbally outline the goals of care, the planned interventions, and what the client is expected to do. Informed

client decision making necessitates awareness of the care plan.

The health-care team

Verbal and written communication
among members of the health-care team is
essential to good care delivery. The written
care plan gives all team members specific
directions concerning what is being striven
for and what to do to provide individualized
care. Verbal communication provides the
health-care team the opportunity to contin-
uously collaborate on improving and ad-
justing care delivery.

Documenting the care plan

Although care plan forms vary in format,
the same principles for documenting apply.
Overall discharge goals are written above
the care plan; nursing diagnoses are identified; long-term and short-term goals are
given for each nursing diagnosis; interventions are entered for each short-term goal;
and the entire care plan is dated and signed.

Correctly written, interventions give precise directions for individualized care delivery. They must be safe and therapeutic, consistent with the care plan, realistic, and specific.

Safe and *therapeutic* interventions protect the client from injury and provide a physical and emotional environment that promotes health maintenance or restoration. The rationale required in student care plans is designed to ensure this. Although the rationale is omitted in professional care plans to save space, the nurse is expected to base all interventions on sound scientific principles.

Every intervention must be *consistent* with all parts of the care plan. Each nursing order must be congruent with the other treatment modalities planned. Interventions should be compatible and complementary. Furthermore, the interventions, taken as a whole, should develop those behaviors or responses specified in the expected outcomes.

Realistic interventions are those that can be implemented, that is, necessary equipment and resources must be available; the personnel must be competent to perform the interventions; and the client must be willing to comply. The planned interventions must be within the legal and educational scope of nursing practice and in agreement with facility policy.

Specific nursing orders are individualized to the particular client and give exact directions as to what to do. Action verbs clearly communicating the expected activity should be used. Examples of precise verbs for each type of nursing intervention follow.

Management

adjust	increase	remove
aspirate	insert	reposition
assist	irrigate	restrain
decrease	maintain	restrict
empty	measure	suction
give	perform	turn
help	provide	weigh

Psychosocial

allow	discuss	share
anticipate	encourage	suggest
counsel	promote	talk

Education

demonstrate	guide	reinforce
discuss	inform	review
educate	instruct	show
explain	list	tell

Consultation

ask	consult	request
collaborate	discuss	share
confer	refer	

Observation

assess	examine	observe
auscultate	measure	palpate
check	monitor	percuss
evaluate	note	watch

In addition to including an action verb the nursing order should specify exactly what and how much. The verb tells what to do, and the noun and modifying clause tell how to do it. For the sake of clarity and brevity standard terminology and accepted abbreviations should be used.

Example

Verb—Irrigate
Noun—Nasogastric tube
Modifier—30 cc normal saline every 2 hours

The intervention would be written as follows:

Irrigate NGT with 30 cc NS q2h

In outline form the care plan looks like the following:

Discharge Goal
Date

Care Plan
Nursing diagnosis 1
 LTG
 STG 1
  Interventions

STG 2
Interventions
Nursing diagnosis 2
LTG
STG 1
Interventions
STG 2
Interventions
Signature

Date

There may be as many nursing diagnoses, expected outcomes, and interventions as necessary to identify and meet the client's needs.

Health-care team collaboration

The care plan is not a static document: it can and should be altered whenever the client's status changes. Nursing diagnoses, expected outcomes, and interventions can be added or discontinued. Daily updating of the care plan reflects effective health-care team communication.

Sharing information about the client's current condition and responses keeps the health-care team up to date. Frequent collaboration decreases the chances of misunderstandings. When all team members have input, the care plan will be comprehensive and pertinent to client needs.

SUMMARY

Care planning is based on the client assessment and the identified nursing diagnoses. During the planning step expected outcomes are established and specific interventions are selected. The care plan is then written and entered into the client's medical record.

Expected outcomes are precise statements that are written in the future tense and describe the desired client response after implementation of the care plan. The discharge goal describes the anticipated condition of the client and to where the client will be discharged. The long-term goal predicts resolution of the problem portion of the nursing diagnosis. Short-term goals are sequential objectives for alleviating the etiology of the problem. When properly written all goals are client centered, singular, observable, measurable, time limited, mutual, and realistic.

Interventions are decided on after the short-term goals have been established. The five types of nursing practice (management, psychosocial care, education, consultation, and observaton) are selected according to the needs and acuity of the problem. The methods for generating and choosing interventions are thinking, researching, and collaborating with the health-care team and the client.

Communication of the care plan involves discussing it with the client, documenting it in the medical record, and conferring frequently with involved members of the health-care team.

The care plan must be specific and individualized to the client. Since the nurse who writes the care plan will not be providing client care around the clock throughout the client's admission, the care plan serves as the major means of communicating the focus of and the actual directions for care delivery. In short it is the instrument by which continuity of care is ensured.

BIBLIOGRAPHY

Alfaro R: Application of nursing process: a step-by-step guide, Philadelphia, 1986, JB Lippincott Co.

American Nurses' Association: Standards of nursing practice, Kansas City, Mo, 1976, The Association.

Atkinson LD and Murray ME: Understanding the nursing process, ed 6, New York, 1988, Macmillan Publishing Co.

Auger JR: Behavioral systems and nursing, Englewood Cliffs, NJ, 1976, Prentice Hall.

Brunner LS and Suddarth DS: Textbook of medical-surgical nursing, ed 6, Philadelphia, 1988, JB Lippincott Co.

Calvillo E: Personal communication, June 4, 1987.

Henderson V: The nature of nursing, New York, 1966, Macmillan Publishing Co.

Iyer PW, Taptich BJ, and Bernocchi-Losey D: Nursing process and nursing diagnosis, Philadelphia, 1986, WB Saunders Co.

Kozier B and Erb G: Fundamentals of nursing: concepts and procedures, ed 3, Menlo Park, Calif, 1987, Addison-Wesley Publishing Co, Inc.

Levin S: Self-care: an emerging component of the health care system, Hosp Health Serv Admin 23:17, 1978.

Linde BJ and Janz NM: Effect of a teaching program on knowledge and compliance of cardiac patients, Nursing Res 28:282, 1979.

Nursing85 Books: Practices, Springhouse, Pa, 1985, Springhouse Corp.

Pender N: Values clarification: health promotion in nursing practice, New York, 1982, Appleton-Century-Crofts.

Prescott PA, Dennis KE, and Jacox AK: Clinical decision making of staff nurses, Image 19:56, 1987.

Redman BK: The process of patient education, ed 6, St Louis, 1988, The CV Mosby Co.

Steiger NJ and Lipson JG: Self-care nursing: theory and practice, Bowie, Md, 1985, Brady Communications Co, Inc.

Watson PM: Patient education: the adult with cancer, Nurs Clin North Am 17:739, 1982.

NURSING CARE PLAN

Discharge Goal:

ASSESSMENT	NURSING DIAGNOSIS
Subjective data Interview	Problem related to etiology

Objective data
  Physical examination
  Health record
  Observation of behavior
  Other sources
 	
Data organization
	Problem—Client response to illness and medical treatment
	
	Etiology—Causative or associated factor(s) within scope of nursing practice

EXPECTED OUTCOMES	INTERVENTIONS	EVALUATION
LTGs in regard to problem	Types	
	Management	
	Psychosocial	
STGs in regard to etiology	Education	
	Consultation	
	Observation	
Criteria		
Patient centered		
Singular		
Observable		
Measurable		
Time limited		
Mutual		
Realistic		

5

Implementation

- **Preparation**
- **Intervention**
- **Documentation**

"Nursing is the diagnosis and treatment of human responses to actual or potential health problems" (American Nurses' Association, 1980). Treatment is the focus of the implementation step of the nursing process. After all preparatory steps are completed, planned interventions are initiated. During the implementation step the care plan is transformed from idea to practice.

The three phases of implementation are (1) preparation, (2) intervention, and (3) communication.

PREPARATION

The entire nursing process up to this point has prepared for the actual treatment of the client. The client's abilities, needs, fears, and hopes have been identified during the assessment and planning steps. The data have been analyzed and nursing diagnoses formulated during the diagnostic step. Goals have been set and interventions to assist the client's return to wellness have been selected during the planning step. The nurse must make the following preparations:

1. Reviewing and prioritizing interventions
2. Organizing resources and care delivery
3. Taking measures to maximize client benefit
4. Recognizing any potential complications

Reviewing and prioritizing

The nursing process is not a static series of steps to be followed in an exclusive sequential order; it is a dynamic process that involves continuous interaction among the steps. The process may proceed out of sequence at times, or several of the steps may occur simultaneously.

The carefully designed care plan requires continual review and reassessment to verify that it is current and appropriate. This reexamination should occur before and after implementing interventions. As the client's status changes, so should the care plan. Additions and deletions are made, and problems and interventions are adjusted and reprioritized.

To make sure the care plan is current and appropriate, the nurse should complete a focused client assessment, review recent nurse's notes, physician's progress notes, and other pertinent sections of the chart, and confer with those members of the health-care team who have had recent client contact. These actions give the nurse an updated overview of client status. Informed judgments about the care plan can then be made.

Reviewing the care plan also allows the nurse to examine the priorities of care, what specific actions need to be taken, what equipment and skills are needed, and who is best qualified to deliver this care. This analysis brings the nurse to the next preparatory phase: organization.

Organizing resources and care delivery

A facility's resources include both equipment and skilled personnel. Organization of equipment and personnel makes efficient, skilled client care possible. Once a plan is determined, the nurse prepares the necessary supplies and decides on the time and provider of care.

Equipment

Most nursing procedures, from bed making to client teaching, require equipment or supplies. The nurse must analyze each planned intervention for needed items. Realistic interventions call for only those things that are available in the facility.

All necessary supplies should be gathered and put in a convenient location, usually where they will be used, before implementing the interventions. The collection of supplies should include any extras that may be needed in case of foreseeable mishaps. Extra sterile gloves, for example, anticipate the possibility of a break in sterile technique. The thorough nurse also arranges the supplies in the order in which they will be used.

Personnel

Nursing care delivery systems vary among facilities and must be taken into account when allocating resources. The system by which nursing is organized determines how personnel are designated for client care delivery. The most common types of nursing delivery systems are the following:

1. Functional
2. Team
3. Case load
4. Primary

Three categories of functions are inherent to professional nursing practice: actual client care, delegation, and coordination. These functions assume varying levels of importance, depending on the nursing system in use.

Functional nursing divides client care into a series of tasks, each of which is delegated to the lowest level of personnel having the requisite skill and competence to complete the task. Each staff member then performs this same task for all clients on the unit. The client is cared for by a number of people who concentrate on their own particular assignments. Advantages of functional nursing are efficiency, economy, and easy organization. The disadvantage is fragmentation of client care; the client is unsure who his or her nurse is. No one person has an overview of the client's status and care plan. Continuity of care is haphazard at best.

Delegating tasks and coordinating personnel become primary functions for the nurse when functional nursing is used. The nurse in charge of the unit must know the competency level of each staff member. Coordination requires good communication to make certain all client care tasks are completed. Special care must be taken to receive reports from each staff member on each client. Maintaining current information on client status in the perspective of the care plan may be difficult, since the emphasis is on tasks not client needs. Good organizational and communication skills are essential for the nurse when delegating and coordinating client care under this system.

Team nursing is a method of care delivery in which a small group of personnel, supervised by a professional nurse, delivers care to a number of clients. The team leader is responsible for the client and the care plan and is in charge of delegating client care to individual team members and coordinating the team's efforts. Cooperation and collaboration are hallmarks of good team nursing.

Advantages of this system include less fragmented and more individualized client care; the client is aware of who is responsible for his or her care. Continuity of care is possible, especially when team composition and assignments are stable. Disadvantages stem primarily from weak leadership skills on the part of the team leader. Team nursing easily deteriorates to the functional level when delegation, coordination, and collaboration are poorly executed.

Team members should be assigned individual client care rather than tasks to be completed for all the team's clients. Team coordination involves making team members available to assist fellow members as needed and planning time for team conferences. Collaboration in the form of reports and team conferences ensure meeting client needs and updating care plans.

Case load nursing, or total client care, is a system in which a nurse is responsible for the complete care of a number of clients throughout a shift. Client care is totally individualized; the nurse assigned to the client is responsible for direct client care, coordination with other departments for services the client is receiving, and the care plan.

Advantages of this care system include an increased awareness of client status and needs and the elimination of fragmented, task-oriented care. Disadvantages become apparent when a nurse is not assigned to the same clients on a regular basis. Continuity of care can be jeopardized when client assignments are changed, since each nurse works autonomously, and collaboration is minimal. Direct client care is emphasized in case load nursing. The total client care nurse provides all aspects of care during the shift. When assigning case loads the unit manager should assign nurses to the same clients to ensure continuity of care. Delegation does not occur under this system; the nurse on each shift independently gives care and is responsible for the care plan.

Primary nursing and total client care are similar, with the exception of duration of responsibility. The primary nurse is responsible for all aspects of the client's care around the clock, from admission to discharge. When the primary nurse is off duty, an associate nurse assumes care of the client. If a problem arises, the associate contacts the primary nurse, who retains full authority and responsibility for decision making.

Major advantage of the primary nursing delivery system is that the primary and associate nurses are experts about the client, and therefore the highest quality and continuity of care can be given. Disadvantages are debatable. Initially, personnel costs are increased, since an all-professional staff is required. Recent studies indicate, however, that primary nursing may be cost effective over the long term, since the higher quality of care results in fewer complications and shortened hospital stays.

In primary nursing client care delegation and coordination are important functions. The primary nurse formulates the care plan, delivers client care, delegates care to associate nurses on the other shifts, and coordinates activities with the associate nurses to ensure continuity of care within the framework of the care plan.

Whatever the nursing care delivery system, careful assignment of staff is of utmost importance. Continuity of individualized care is a primary consideration when organizing personnel for client care.

Maximizing client benefit

The client receives optimal benefit from nursing actions when the nurse takes time to prepare both the environment and the client before intervening.

The environment

Client care does not happen in a vacuum. Environmental factors influence both the delivery and the reception of care. The surroundings in which nursing activities occur should be safe and conducive to achieving the particular goal of the intervention strategy. Safety is always the nurse's first concern. If the client has sensory deficits or an alteration in level of consciousness, the environment must be arranged to prevent injury. Special rooms, rearrangement of furniture and equipment, and provision for additional personnel are examples of creating safe surroundings.

The client benefits most from nursing interventions when the surroundings are compatible with the activities. Privacy promotes relaxation when body parts are exposed. Reducing distractions enhances learning opportunities. Provision of adequate warmth and lighting prevents intrusion of environmental factors.

The client

Before beginning interventions the nurse should make the client as physically and psychologically comfortable as possible. Pain frequently interferes with a client's full concentration and cooperation. Comfort measures or medication for pain before initiating interventions enable the client to participate as desired. If client alertness is needed, the dose of pain medication should be sufficient to relieve discomfort but not impair mental faculties.

Even if pain is not a factor, the client should be physically comfortable during the interventions. Controlling environmental factors, positioning, and taking care of other physical needs should precede initiation of the intervention session. The nurse should also consider the client's level of endurance and plan only the amount of activity that the client can comfortably tolerate.

Awareness of the client's psychosocial needs helps the nurse to create a favorable emotional climate. Some clients feel reassured by having a significant other present to lend encouragement and moral support. Other strategies include planning sufficient time or multiple opportunities for the client to work through and ventilate feelings and anxieties. Adequate preparations allow the client to reap full benefit and alleviate the need for repetitious interventions.

Recognizing potential complications

Risks to the client arise both from the illness itself and from treatment procedures. It is the nurse's respnsibility to identify these risks, evaluate the relative benefit of the treatment versus the risk, and initiate preventive measures.

Many client conditions in and of themselves place the client at risk for additional complications. The nurse's knowledge of pathophysiology helps in the identification of potential problems. Scientific rationales help the nurse evaluate the usefulness of preventive strategies in forestalling problem development. For example, a confused client is at risk for pulmonary complications because of extended periods of immobility.

The nurse knows that getting the client out of bed will expand the bases of the lungs but also realizes that this activity poses a risk to the client's safety. Preventive safety measures may necessitate remaining with the client while the client is out of bed or securing the client in a chair with a posey restraint and checking the client frequently.

Some nursing procedures also pose risks for the client. The nurse needs to be aware of potential complications and institute precautionary measures. For instance, the client receiving tube feedings via nasogastric tube is at risk for aspiration. The nurse should have pharyngeal suction equipment at the bedside before initiating the feedings.

INTERVENTION

The primary focus of the implementation step is intervening on the client's behalf. All efforts to date have been directed to this moment; the care plan is about to become reality.

The following four areas of nursing care are considered when initiating actual nursing interventions:

1. Nursing skills

2. Level of care needed by the client
3. Adjustments required during care delivery
4. Caring

Skills

Nursing practice is composed of cognitive, interpersonal, and technical skills. Each of these skills is required to implement the five kinds of nursing interventions.

Management, although primarily technical in nature, also demands cognitive and interpersonal skills. The nurse must understand the reasons for the procedures and must be able to anticipate and recognize subsequent complications that may result. Because many procedures are unpleasant or uncomfortable, interpersonal skills are invaluable in reassuring and comforting the client who might otherwise be uncooperative.

Psychosocial interventions are mainly interpersonal. They are concerned with two people meeting and working with emotional or relational issues. The technique of psychosocial nursing relies on the ability to use good communication skills and such strategies as behavior modification or crisis intervention. The nurse must have the intellectual competency to assess the client's psychosocial status, to select appropriate intervention techniques, and to evaluate responses accurately.

Client education requires cognitive, interpersonal, and technical skills in equal measure. The nurse must be able to identify learning needs and know the information to be taught. The ability to communicate clearly and at the client's level of understanding is essential. Client teaching often involves physical demonstration of new health-care measures. Technical expertise reassures the client that the skill is readily learnable.

Cognitive and interpersonal skills are most commonly used when initiating consultation interventions. Knowledge of what services the client needs and where to find them is needed. The nurse must then facilitate the referral on both sides with good communication. The client needs to understand what to expect from the referral, and the consulting person or agency needs accurate and concise information to provide the requested assistance.

Observation makes use of all three skills.

The nurse needs sufficient interpersonal skills to avoid giving the impression of curiosity or making the client feel like an object on display. It is important to convey a feeling of caring. Cognitive skills involve knowing what to assess and how to analyze the information, as well as the ability to evaluate client responses objectively. The specialized education of the nurse provides technical information and skills to make accurate and pertinent observations.

While implementing the five types of interventions the nurse must know not only what to do but also how much to do. Assessment of the client and the amount of behavior change desired direct the nurse to the level of care necessary to assist the patient in goal achievement.

Level of care

Even when they have the same medical diagnoses, no two clients are in exactly the same condition or have precisely the same needs, strengths, or weaknesses. Every client must be given care at a level that reflects the individual's precise physical and emotional status and that best

Patient condition:	Incapacitated	Ill	Well
Nursing care:	Total	Assistive	Supportive

Fig. 5. *Continuum of client condition and level of nursing care.*

promotes attainment of expected outcomes. The level of care the nurse provides a client can be thought of as a continuum with the following three basic divisions: (1) total care, (2) assistive care, and (3) supportive care. The continuum of client condition and nursing level of care is illustrated in Figure 5.

Total care

The client who is incapacitated, unconscious, or completely unable to provide self-care requires total nursing care. This means that the nurse maintains bodily functions and provides all nurturing activities until the client improves sufficiently to participate in the care procedures. Total nursing care may extend to all areas of function, as when the client is unconscious. The nurse, in such cases, does everything for the client, including maintaining autonomic functions, such as respiration or blood pressure, as needed. All five types of nursing interventions are used but in a manner that differs from the other levels of care.

Management and observation strategies focus on maintaining life and improving its quality. Consultation is often required for the client who may have several serious problems. Client education is limited to explaining procedures as they are performed, even though the client is unconscious. Psychosocial, educational, and consultative interventions are also implemented for the client's significant others.

Sometimes a client is conscious but is still unable to participate in one or more areas of care; that is, the client is able to provide some self-care but has a total inability to do something(s) adequately. Clients with spinal cord injuries are good examples of this category of infirmity. Suppose a client has a high spinal cord injury and is completely paralyzed. Although retaining both full consciousness and complete use of intellectual powers, the client is unable to care for any bodily needs. Nursing care is total in respect to this client's physical needs. On the other hand the client may only require assistive or supportive levels of care for emotional, intellectual, and social needs. In such an instance total care involves management strategies only; the remaining four kinds of interventions are at a different level.

Assistive care

Most hospitalized clients require an assistive level of care during most of their stay. They are able to provide some of their own care but need help in some aspects. At the assistive level the nurse and the client work together; the nurse supplements the client's capabilities whenever necessary.

This area of the continuum has a wide span, from those clients who require assistance with almost all activity to those who only need it in one or two types of situations. It is the nurse's responsibility to determine what the client can do and the amount and kind of assistance that is required. Assistive care includes all five types of nursing interventions. The focus of care at this level is to decrease or eliminate unhealthy responses and to foster healthy ones. Management and observation strategies are used until the client is capable of normal performance. Educational interventions are aimed at teaching the client to adapt or learn new self-care activities. Psychosocial and consultative measures are concentrated on adding to the client's psychologic and social assets.

The surgical client provides a ready example of one who needs assistive care. During the immediate postoperative period the client requires assistance with almost everything. Generally, recovery is rapid, and the client daily needs less and less assistance with normal activities. However, the nurse may still perform all the dressing changes or other technical procedures. In the meantime the nurse is also using psychosocial and educative measures to assist the client in adapting to a new body image and in learning new health-care information. The nurse may also confer with the family or make a referral to a home health agency for post-discharge care.

The assistive level of care changes frequently for almost all clients. Ongoing assessment is necessary to make sure that the level of care is compatible with the client's capabilities. As care is given, the client's condition should improve, and the amount of needed assistance should lessen. The client should progress to the supportive level of care.

Supportive care

Some clients are physically capable of providing their own care but have difficulty doing so because of either a lack of knowledge or motivation. At this level of care the client actually performs all health-care measures while the nurse teaches, supports, and guides.

Psychosocial counseling and teaching are the primary intervention modes. The client may need information and support for decision making or may need anticipatory guidance or emotional support during grief work. Perhaps motivational reinforcement is required. Clients in clinics and physicians' offices often use the nurse as a consultative resource. Nursing observations are limited to assessing the client's continued need for supportive care. The client should soon be self-sufficient. Termination of the helping relationship should be planned and gradual, but it should occur before the client becomes dependent.

As interventions are implemented, the

client's condition and responses should improve. Thus client needs and the level of nursing care should also change, necessitating adjustments in the level, kind, and amount of nursing strategies.

Adjustments

As discussed previously the client's condition must be frequently assessed and the level of care adjusted accordingly. The amount of nursing assistance provided for each concern should be reevaluated on a daily basis.

Client responses while the interventions are being implemented may also indicate the need for an adjustment. Any negative reaction is cause for evaluating the appropriateness of the intervention. An intervention may appear unsuitable for a variety of reasons. Perhaps the client had insufficient preparation. Maybe an important factor, such as a hearing loss, was overlooked when the intervention was planned. The client may be preoccupied with another worry. If an intervention is not going smoothly, the nurse needs to pause, reassess the situation, and consider whether changes are needed. The care plan is flexible; it is meant to be altered whenever the client's status changes.

Caring

Nursing is described as an art and a science. So far this text has dealt with the more scientific aspect, that is, the planning and provision of care based on reason and scientific principles. The other side of nursing is nurturance. It has to do with human meeting human. It involves sensitivity, understanding, caring, compassion, and respect.

The two faces of nursing go hand in hand; if one is missing, nursing has not been fulfilled. Caring without competence is malpractice; technical perfection without caring is inhumane.

The nurse is legally responsible and accountable for providing technically correct care and therefore can be legally prosecuted for providing incompetent care (malpractice) or failing to provide competent care (negligence). Professional and ethical standards require the nurse to go beyond competence to caring. No law mandates the art of nursing, no law but the higher laws of professional commitment and the nurse's own conscience.

COMMUNICATION

Ongoing communication with the client and the health-care team and accurate documentation are crucial for continued quality care delivery. Good communication forms the basis for objective evaluation.

The client

Since the client is the focus of the interventions, the client should be the first person with whom the nurse should communicate. During and after intervening the nurse assesses the client's response and judges the effectiveness of the interventions. Equally important is the client's view. Does the client think the interventions are helpful or effective? Does the client have any complaints or suggestions? Seeking the client's input helps keep interventions pertinent and individualized. It also adds the client's point of view to the data to be evaluated.

The health-care team

All implemented interventions and the resulting client responses are communicated to the health-care team through verbal reports and written documentation in the client's chart. Neither type of communication by itself is sufficient; both methods are essential to continuity of care.

Reporting

Reporting is the verbal communication of specific information about the client to another member or group of members of the health-care team. Reports should be short and concise and include only relevant data. They should be factual and specific as to what, when, and how much. Two times when nurses ordinarily give reports are to the physician, when the client has an untoward response, and to the oncoming nurse or team at the end of the shift.

Reports to physicians require good nursing judgment. If the physician orders the reporting of test results, no question exists; that is, the nurse notifies the physician when the results arrive, giving the exact information requested. Nursing judgment becomes a factor when no report is ordered and the client experiences an unusual or unexpected reaction. The nurse must then consider the importance of the new data relevant to the client's status and medical treatment. The decision to report is based on the nurse's knowledge of pathophysiology, treatment parameters, and the client's condition. If the nurse has any doubts about the implications for client welfare, the physician should be notified.

When calling the physician the nurse identifies the facility, the client's name and medical diagnosis, and the reason for the call. The nurse should avoid making statements such as "I was wondering" or "I have a hunch" and should instead present facts and objective data. Test results, vital signs, and other information the physician may inquire about should be readily available. The report should be factual and organized.

Change-of-shift reports take several forms: some are audio taped, and others are given in person, either on a nurse-to-nurse or nurse-to-team basis. The tape recorded report is usually brief, but it does not afford the oncoming nurse the opportunity to ask questions. The nurse-to-nurse report allows for questions, but complications can arise when client-load assignments differ on the two shifts. The nurse-to-team report also allows for questions but can be time consuming if all oncoming nurses are required to listen to reports on all clients.

Information to report at the change of shift remains the same regardless of the reporting method. All information should be as quantitative as possible. The following should be included for every client:

1. Identifying data—Name, age, sex, and room and bed number
2. Medical identification—Medical diagnosis and physician(s)
3. Medical treatments—Diagnostic tests and results and therapies and responses
4. Physical status—Pertinent physical assessment data and significant changes or problems
5. Psychosocial status—Emotional responses, information needs, and significant changes or problems
6. Nursing concerns—Care plan status, what has been accomplished, what needs to be done, current concerns, and helpful hints to facilitate meeting client needs

Receiving a report is as active a process as giving it. If information is missing, it is the receiving nurse's responsibility to ask questions. Complete reports save nursing time and ensure coordinated care.

Documentation

Recording is the last phase of the implementation step. Despite the seemingly endless variety of forms only two basic systems are used to organize medical records: the source-oriented record and the problem-oriented record.

The *source-oriented* system of recording divides the medical record into sections according to who provides the service. Each discipline has its own section; the physician section includes physician's orders, progress notes, and history and physical data; nursing has a progress notes section; laboratory has a section for results, as do other departments. Each discipline records only in its own section. The advantage of this system is that each section is easy to locate. The disadvantage is that information about a specific problem is difficult to locate, since it is scattered throughout the chart.

Nursing has several forms on which it records: the nursing admission sheet, medication records, flowsheets, and the nurses' notes. Upon the client's arrival on the unit the admitting nurse completes the admission sheet, which usually includes demographic data, a brief history, and an initial physical assessment. Every time a medication is given, the nurse records it on the medication sheet. Flowsheets provide a graphic record of routine care and regular client assessments, such as vital signs and intake and output. Nursing progress notes are recorded chronologically in narrative style. All assessments, interventions, and evaluations are documented as they occur. Frequency of charting depends on the client's condition and the facility's policy. All documents are dated and signed.

The *problem-oriented* system (POR or POMR) arranges data in a manner similar to the nursing process. Client problems are the focus, and documentation from each discipline is integrated throughout the chart. This system makes client problem information readily accessible and facilitates team coordination of care. Four major sections of this system are the data base, the problem list, the care plan, and the progress notes.

The data base includes admission assessments from all the disciplines involved with the client. It has standardized forms for each discipline. Demographic data, history, physical, diagnostic studies, social, and family information are recorded here. The collected data form the basis for the problem list.

The problem list identifies client problems as analyzed from the data base by each discipline. Each problem is numbered sequentially. The number identifies the problem and the order in which it was added to the list, but it does not indicate the problem's priority. This list is usually placed at the front of the chart for ready access by all team members. Problems are added and discontinued as the client's status changes.

The care plan for each problem is formulated by the person who identifies it. Each plan is assigned the same number as its corresponding problem. Space is available for entering expected outcomes, interventions, and evaluation dates. The plan is comprehensive; it includes the care plan from each participating discipline. It is usually located at the front of the chart, directly behind the problem list.

Multidisciplinary progress notes document the client's progress for the problem identified. Each entry is begun by writing the problem and care plan number. The format for all disciplines is structured according to *s*ubjective data, *o*bjective data, *a*nalysis, and *p*lan, or SOAP. Some agencies use the variations SOAPIE or SOAPIER, reflecting the addition of *i*ntervention, *e*valuation, and *r*evision. A few differences can be found in the content of some sections of the SOAP note, depending on whether a problem is being opened, continued, or discontinued.

Example

Opening a new problem

S—Client statement about problem or symptoms

O—Objective data that substantiates both the problem and the etiology of the nursing diagnosis; includes data from the four assessment sources

A—Problem r/t etiology, No. __ (formal statement of the nursing diagnosis)

P—Initiate care plan No. __

The nursing diagnosis is numbered and entered on the problem list, and the care plan is documented on the care plan page. All three entries are dated and signed.

Example

Continuing a problem

S—Client statement

O—Updated observations on the client's condition relative to the problem and etiology; responses to interventions

A—Evaluation of status of the problem: improving, worsening, or no change

P—Continue with nursing orders; add new or revised nursing interventions.

Nursing orders added in a progress note are not appended to the initial care plan but are considered part of the progressive care plan. Frequency of charting depends on the client's condition.

Example

Discontinuing a problem

S—Client statement

O—Objective assessments indicating resolution of the problem and etiology

A—Problem No. __ resolved

P—Discontinue problem; monitor for recurrence

The problem and corresponding care plan are then discontinued (dc) on the problem list and care plan pages. Yellowing out or writing "dc" and the date are the usual methods of discontinuing an entry.

If the agency uses the SOAPIE or SOAPIER format, the progression is the same, with the following additions:

I— List of interventions completed

E— Evaluation of client response to each intervention

R— Revision or reassessment of any or all components: diagnosis, goals, interventions

Discharge and transfer summaries list the client's continuing problems, their status, and the care plan. They can be written in a narrative style or according to the SOAP format, whereby each problem is charted in a separate SOAP note or combined in one SOAP note, with each problem numbered in each section. Each facility has its own policy as to which method is preferred.

SUMMARY

The implementation step is the action-oriented phase of the nursing process in which the care plan becomes care. The three stages of the implementation step are preparation, intervention, and communication.

The nurse prepares to intervene by reviewing and prioritizing interventions, organizing supplies and personnel, preparing the client and environment, and anticipating and preventing potential complications.

Interventions require cognitive, interpersonal, and technical skills. When implementing care the nurse must consider what level of care will result in optimal client benefit. The selection of total, assistive, or supportive care is based on the client's condition and capabilities. As the client's condition changes, interventions and level of care are adjusted accordingly. Nursing care, often technical in nature, must always be tempered by human compassion and respect.

Communication of completed interventions and client responses is both an oral and written process. Reports are made to the physician and during the change of shift. Documentation of the client's progress is done in the progress notes. In the source-oriented system the nurse's notes are chronologically recorded in a narrative format. Problem-oriented progress notes are written in the SOAP format.

The implementation step is the focal point of the nursing process. It is what nursing is about: nursing care delivery. When properly planned and implemented the implementation step resolves client problems and assists the client back to health. Accurate documentation of interventions sets the stage for objective evaluation of goal achievement.

BIBLIOGRAPHY

American Nurses' Association: Nursing: a social policy statement, Kansas City, Mo, 1980, The Association.

Arndt C and Huckabay LMD: Nursing administration: theory for practice with a systems approach, ed 2, St Louis, 1980, The CV Mosby Co.

Brunner LS and Suddarth DS: Textbook of medical-surgical nursing, ed 6, Philadelphia, 1988, JB Lippincott Co.

Davis AJ and Aroskar MA: Ethical dilemmas and nursing practice, ed 2, Norwalk, Conn, 1983, Appleton-Century-Crofts.

Grubbs J: The Johnson behavioral system model. In Riehl JP and Roy C, editors: Conceptual models for nursing practice, ed 2, New York, 1980, Appleton-Century-Crofts.

Iyer PW, Taptich BJ, and Bernocchi-Losey D: Nursing process and nursing diagnosis, Philadelphia, 1986, WB Saunders Co.

Kozier B and Erb G: Fundamentals of nursing: concepts and procedures, ed 3, Menlo Park, Calif, 1987, Addison-Wesley Publishing Co, Inc.

Luckman J and Sorensen KC: Medical-surgical nursing: a psychophysiologic approach, ed 3, 1987, WB Saunders Co.

Nursing85 Books: Practices, Springhouse, Pa, 1985, Springhouse Corp.

Orem DE: Nursing: concepts of practice, ed 2, New York, 1980, McGraw-Hill, Inc.

Roy C: Introduction to nursing: an adaptation model, Englewood Cliffs, NJ, 1976, Prentice Hall.

NURSING CARE PLAN

Discharge Goal:

ASSESSMENT	NURSING DIAGNOSIS
Subjective data Interview	Problem related to etiology
	Problem—Client response to

Objective data
    Physical exam-
      ination
	illness or medical treat-
	ment

Health record
    Observation of
      behavior
    Other sources
	Etiology—Causative or asso-
	ciated factor(s) within
	scope of nursing practice

Data organization	

EXPECTED OUTCOMES	INTERVENTIONS	EVALUATION
LTG in regard to problem	Types Management Psychosocial Education Consultation Observation	
STGs in regard to etiology		
Criteria Client centered Singular Observable Measurable Time limited Mutual Realistic	Phases Preparation Intervention Communication	

6

Evaluation

- ■ *Evaluation of goal achievement*
- ■ *Revision of care plan*
- ■ *Documentation*

Evaluation, the fifth and last step of the nursing process, is either a terminal or a recycling step. Up to now the client has been assessed, problems diagnosed, and a care plan formulated and implemented. During evaluation the nurse judges the success of these steps by examining the client's responses and comparing them with the behavior stated in the expected outcomes. The results of the comparison determine whether the process will be terminated or reactivated.

When the nursing process is reactivated, each step is reconsidered for currentness, accuracy, and appropriateness. Needed revisions are made and implemented; these are then evaluated in turn. The sequence is cyclical until the problem is resolved.

The three phases of the evaluation step are (1) evaluation of goal achievement, (2) care plan revision, and (3) communication of results.

EVALUATION OF GOAL ACHIEVEMENT

The overall purpose of nursing care is to assist the client in resolving health problems. Evaluation of goal achievement is the determination of whether this purpose was accomplished. This determination is made by matching the client's behavior or physiologic response and the behavior or response specified in the expected outcome.

There are degrees of goal attainment. If the client's response exactly matches or exceeds the goal criteria, the goal is met. If the client's behavior is beginning to show change but does not yet completely meet the specified criteria, the goal is partially met. If there is no progress whatsoever, the goal is not met. If the goal is correctly stated, the nurse can determine precisely how well the goal was met. To evaluate objectively the degree of the client's success in achieving a goal, the nurse should use the following steps:

1. *Examine* the goal statement to identify the exact desired client behavior or response.
2. *Assess* the client for presence of that behavior or response.
3. *Compare* the established goal criteria with the client's behavior or response.
4. *Judge* the degree of agreement between goal criteria and the client's behavior or response.

Example

Expected outcome   Will sit in chair at bedside for 15 min on 7/8.

Client behavior assessment   Sat in chair at bedside for 20 min on 7/8.

Comparison

Goal criteria	Client behavior
Sit in chair	Accomplished
Chair at bedside	Accomplished
For 15 min	Exceeded
On 7/8	Accomplished

Judgment   Client met or exceeded all criteria of expected outcome. Goal met.

Short-term goals

Short-term goals are statements of progressive behavioral steps the client needs to accomplish to modify or remove the etiology of the problem. By definition they have short time frames, encompassing as few as one or two intervention sessions.

After the specified interval, or when all interventions listed for that short-term goal have been completed, the nurse evaluates the client's ability to demonstrate the behavior or response stated in the goal statement. Evaluation after each short-term goal is essential because of the sequential nature of goals; each lays the groundwork for the next. Failure to evaluate each short-term goal makes it difficult to determine where the sequence faltered.

If the client achieves the short-term goal, the nurse continues with the care plan. If the nurse's evaluation determines that the short-term goal was not met or only partially met, the nurse activates the process of reassessment and revision.

The evaluation statement should specify exactly the client behavior or response that led to the judgment about the goal's status. For example, the nursing diagnosis "Potential alteration in health maintenance related to lack of knowledge in regard to identification and management of infection" might have the following as a short-term goal:

By 6/2 will identify redness, heat, swelling, and pain at incision site as signs of infection.
Evaluation of STG
Met
On 6/2 stated redness, heat, pain, and swelling at incision site are signs of infection
Partially met
On 6/2 identified only redness and pain as signs of infection
Not met
On 6/2 stated lack of knowledge concerning what to look for as a sign of infection at incision site

Long-term goals

A long-term goal specifies the behavior or response indicating problem resolution. It is the end result of the etiology being altered or removed as a consequence of short-term goal achievement. The long-term goal is therefore evaluated at the completion of all short-term goals for a nursing diagnosis. The diagnosis "Alteration in electrolyte bal-

ance related to loss of gastric secretions"
would be evaluated as follows:

LTG
Electrolytes will be within normal limits
(WNL) by 8/8.
Evaluation of LTG
Met
K^+: 4.2, Cl^-: 102, and Na^+: 140 on 8/8;
all electrolytes WNL
Partially met
K^+: 3.0, Cl^-: 102, and Na^+: 140 on 8/8;
remains hypokalemic; Na^+ and Cl^-
WNL.
Not met
K^+: 3.0, Cl^-: 95, and Na^+: 148 on 8/8;
remains hypokalemic, hypochloremic,
and hypernatremic

Discharge goals

The discharge goal (DCG) concerns the
client's overall condition at the time of discharge from the facility. It encompasses the
status of all identified nursing diagnoses and
looks to the client's ability to manage health
care after discharge.

Example

DCG
Discharge home with life-style changes
Nursing Diagnoses

1. Alteration in electrolyte balance related to loss of gastric secretions
2. Potential alteration in health maintenance related to lack of knowledge in regard to identification and management of infection
3. Body image disturbance related to acceptance of ileostomy

When preparing the client for discharge the nurse should evaluate the status of each nursing diagnosis. Perhaps problem No. 1 is resolved; problem No. 2 is partially resolved; and problem No. 3 is unresolved. In such a case evaluation of the discharge goal would indicate that the client is physically ready for discharge but requires a referral for further assistance in developing a new body image that will foster learning new health management practices. Final evaluation of the discharge goal would then state the following:

Discharge goal partially met; referral to home health agency made for continued assistance with health maintenance and body image concerns.

CARE PLAN REVISION

After the goals have been evaluated, adjustments are made to the care plan as indicated by the evaluated status of the goals. If a goal was met, that portion of the care plan is discontinued. Not met and partially met goals reactivate the nursing process sequence. Following reassessment, modification of nursing diagnoses, expected outcomes, and interventions are made as needed. At this point evaluation becomes concurrent with each step of the process.

Discontinuing

When short-term or long-term goals are evaluated as having been achieved, the nurse should confirm this evaluation with the client. If both are in agreement that the objectives have been met, the nurse then discontinues that portion of the care plan. Revisions indicating short-term goal or problem resolution provide documentary evidence of improvement in the client's condition. This is the aim of nursing care; it indicates the client no longer requires nursing assistance in this area.

Modification

The process of evaluation involves identifying those variables, or factors, that interfered with goal achievement. Usually a change in the client's condition, needs, or abilities makes alteration of the care plan necessary.

Lack of goal achievement may also result from an error in nursing judgment or a misstep along the nursing process. Clients frequently present very complex situations and problems. The nurse should always keep in mind the possibility of inadvertently overlooking or misjudging something. Whenever there is failure to achieve a goal, no matter what the reason, the entire nursing process sequence is reactivated to discover what changes need to be made to promote, maintain, or restore the client's health.

Reassessment

A complete reassessment of all client factors relating to the problem and etiology is the first step in reactivating the process. As in the original assessment data are collected from all available sources. The nurse should be particularly alert for changes in the client's status.

Reassessment ensures the data base is accurate and current. It may also reveal the missing link, that is, the critical piece of new information that may have been previously overlooked, thus interferring with goal achievement. All new data are sorted, evaluated for changes or differences from the original data base, and documented.

The following is an example of a reassessment that reveals new data. A client, who was originally assessed as anxious and lacking information about a procedure, might be reassessed as remaining anxious. However, the reassessment might also reveal that the client is no longer anxious because of a lack of knowledge. Now the client is anxious because of potential complications that may result from the procedure. The changed cause of the anxiety requires a different nursing diagnosis.

Nursing diagnoses

After the client has been reassessed, all nursing diagnoses are evaluated in light of the new data. Is the diagnostic statement accurately worded for the present situation? Is the problem current? Are the etiologic factors still operative? The problem list should then be revised to reflect the client's current status. A new problem may be diagnosed. If a previous diagnosis no longer accurately reflects the problem, it should be discontinued and the modified statement entered. It is far more important that the list of nursing diagnoses be accurate than that the problem list be short. As the client's condition changes, so will the diagnoses.

To continue the example presented under "Reassessment," the original nursing diagnosis would have been "Anxiety related to lack of knowledge about thoracentesis." As a result of the change in the cause of the anxiety, the nursing diagnosis would be revised as "Anxiety related to concern in regard to potential postthoracentesis complications." The different etiology mandates revision of short-term goals and interventions.

Expected outcomes

Every goal, long term and short term, should be inspected for needed changes. Even the goals for those nursing diagnoses that remained unchanged during the evaluation process should be examined for appropriateness. Ascertaining that each goal is realistic for the problem, etiology, and time frame is particularly important. Unrealistic expected behaviors and time frames make goal achievement very difficult.

Expected outcomes for new or revised nursing diagnoses should be written. When the goal is still appropriate but has not yet been met, the evaluation date may need to be changed to allow more time. All goals should reflect the current focus of care and realistic expectations for client achievement.

Continuing the example, a short-term goal for the original etiology (lack of knowledge about thoracentesis) may be the following:

After the first teaching session client will state understanding of the purpose of the thoracentesis.

This goal would be irrelevant to the revised etiology (concern in regard to potential postthoracentesis complications). A new short-term goal might read as follows:

After first teaching session client will state importance of not moving during procedure to reduce risk of pneumothorax.

The new short-term goal would then indicate the need for different teaching interventions.

Interventions

The evaluation of interventions must examine two aspects: the appropriateness of the interventions selected and the implementation process.

Upon evaluation it may be determined that some planned interventions are designed for an inappropriate level of nursing care. If the level of care needs to be changed, a different action verb, such as "assist" in place of "provide," may be substituted.

Sometimes the level of care is appropriate, but the interventions themselves are unsuitable because of a change in the short-term goal. The interventions should be discontinued and new ones planned.

In the continuing example the interventions for teaching the purpose of thoracentesis would be discontinued. New interventions instructing the client how to participate in preventing complications would be added.

During implementation the nurse assesses the client's response during and immediately after intervening. Evaluation of client response is actually the beginning of the evaluation process. If the response is favorable, the care plan proceeds. Reassessment of implementation occurs when the intervention is evaluated as unsuccessful. The nurse must then examine the other components of the implementation step, such as environmental and client preparation, anticipated complications, or use of personal or technical skills during care delivery.

Modifications in actual implementation strategies should be guided by the nature of the client's unfavorable response. Conferring with other nurses may yield suggestions for improving the approach to care delivery that will be compatible with the client's needs.

Perhaps the nurse, in the example, had mentioned potential complications while teaching the client about thoracentesis. The warning may have generated the client's concern about complications. When planning new educational interventions the nurse should evaluate the client's anxiety level and the teaching method. Interpersonal skills may need to be modified to reassure the client and instill confidence while providing the necessary information.

An error during the care planning and delivery sequence should not be interpreted as nursing inadequacy. The nursing process is a systematic method that eliminates random care delivery and assists the nurse in providing individualized client care. It does not guarantee perfect nursing judgment. In fact, perfection is not expected. The process is structured so that human imperfection is taken into account. That is the reason for the evaluation step.

Evaluation gives the nurse the opportunity to assess success, review the process, and make adjustments and improvements. Thus evaluation is both a safety device for client care enhancement and a means of positive feedback for the nurse.

COMMUNICATION

Communication is an essential part of each step of the nursing process. The client must be consulted, the health-care team notified, and the evaluation statements documented.

The client

The client should be consulted about the quality, quantity, and effectiveness of care. This should occur after each intervention session, especially when evaluating goals, and before discharge. The client's family may also be consulted. Client input is essential to valid evaluation; a goal cannot be considered accomplished or the client adequately prepared for discharge unless the client agrees.

The health-care team

After goal achievement has been evaluated, communication with other members of the health-care team occurs in two forms: conferring and documenting.

Conferring

Oral reports of achieved goals and resolved problems are normally given to the oncoming nurse at the change of shift. The oncoming nurse is thus prepared to validate the evaluation.

When a goal is evaluated as not having been met, the nurse needs to confer with the other members of the team who know the client. Someone may have information that will be useful in care plan revision or have an insight regarding more effective implementation.

Documenting

Both the evaluation of goal achievement and all parts of the care plan revision need to be accurately and fully documented in the progress notes and on the care plan.

If a short-term goal is met, both the goal and the accompanying interventions are discontinued. If the long-term goal for a nursing diagnosis is achieved, that diagnosis and the associated care plan are discontinued. A progress note clearly identifying the behaviors or responses indicating goal achievement must also be written.

Should a long-term or short-term goal be evaluated as not met or only partially met, necessary care plan revisions are made, and a new evaluation date is set. The progress note should specify what behaviors have changed and what remains to be accomplished.

The discharge goal, when evaluated as met, should be noted on the care plan and dated, and then the care plan is discontinued in entirety. The progress note should indicate that all problems are resolved and that the client is prepared for discharge with home-care instructions.

When the client is being discharged and one or more nursing diagnoses remain unresolved, interventions should indicate a referral that will meet the client's continuing needs after discharge. In making the referral the nurse should briefly state the problem and list those life-style changes or physical needs the client still needs to accomplish. The progress note should summarize what has been accomplished and indicate that a referral has been made to follow up on the client's remaining problems.

Quality assurance

Quality assurance is the planned, organized evaluation of the client care provided in a facility. This evaluation rates the efficiency and effectiveness of nursing care based on established standards of care. Care delivery may be evaluated from three viewpoints: structure, process, and outcome.

The evaluation of structure examines the setting in which client care is provided. It includes evaluation of the physical setting and equipment, administrative aspects, and the nursing system in use. The rationale is that a good environment promotes quality care.

Process evaluation looks at the manner in which care is delivered. Each phase of the nursing process and the technical competence of the nursing staff is examined. The quality of care is evaluated on the appropriateness and completeness of care.

Outcome evaluation reviews the end result of care in terms of client recovery and survival. This evaluation is usually expressed in percentages. The assumption is that the quality of care can be measured by the percentage of favorable outcomes.

Quality assurance is becoming an increasingly important factor in nursing care evaluation because of the prospective payment system and the need to validate the effectiveness of professional nursing. Quality nursing, based on accepted standards of care, promotes client health and the advancement of the profession.

SUMMARY

The evaluation step of the nursing process is both a terminal and a recurrent action for the nurse. It is terminal in that goal achievement is evaluated at the end of the nursing process sequence. The recurrent aspect involves the evaluation of each part of the process when goals are not met.

All nursing care is goal directed. Therefore what must be evaluated is the client's attainment of expected outcomes. When all goals have been met, care is terminated. When goals have not been met, the care plan is evaluated and revised to promote goal achievement.

Revision of the care plan depends on the evaluation of each step of the nursing process sequence. Modifications to any portion are made based on changes in client status and focus of care.

Communication of the results of the evaluation of expected outcomes is vital to the quality and continuity of care. The client must concur in the evaluation. Goal evaluation is communicated to the health-care team by reports and by documentation in the health record.

Quality assurance is the evaluation of the efficacy of care delivery by the health-care team. The structure, process, and outcomes of care are measured against established standards of care.

The purpose of the entire nursing process is to maintain and improve the quality of client care. Few human endeavors are more valuable than this desire to improve the well-being of other humans.

BIBLIOGRAPHY

Alfaro R: Application of nursing process: a step-by-step guide, Philadelphia, 1986, JB Lippincott Co.

American Nurses' Association: Standards of nursing practice, Kansas City, Mo, 1973, The Association.

American Nurses' Association: Nursing: a social policy statement, Kansas City, Mo, 1980, The Association.

Carpenito LJ: Nursing diagnoses: application to clinical practice, Philadelphia, 1983, JB Lippincott Co.

Hamric AB and Spross J: The clinical nurse specialist in theory and practice, New York, 1983, Grune & Stratton.

Iyer PW, Taptich BJ, and Bernocchi-Losey D: Nursing process and nursing diagnosis, Philadelphia, 1986, WB Saunders Co.

Kozier B and Erb G: Fundamentals of nursing: concepts and procedures, ed 3, Menlo Park, Calif, 1987, Addison-Wesley Publishing Co, Inc.

Patrick ML et al: Medical-surgical nursing: pathophysiological concepts, Philadelphia, 1986, JB Lippincott Co.

Sechrest L and Cohen RY: Evaluating outcomes in health care. In Stone GC, Cohen F, and Adler NE, editors: Health psychology, San Francisco, 1982, Jossey-Bass, Inc, Publishers.

Tucker SM et al: Patient care standards: nursing process, diagnosis, and outcome, ed 4, St Louis, 1984, The CV Mosby Co.

NURSING CARE PLAN

Discharge Goal:

ASSESSMENT	NURSING DIAGNOSIS
Subjective data 　Interview	Problem related to etiology
Objective data 　Physical exam- 　　ination 　Health record 　Observation of 　　behavior 　Other sources	Problem—Client response to illness or medical treat- ment Etiology—Causative or asso- ciated factor(s) within scope of nursing practice
Data organization	

EXPECTED OUTCOMES	INTERVENTIONS	EVALUATION

LTG in regard to problem	Types
	  Management
	  Psychosocial
		Goal achievement
		  STGs
		  LTGs

STGs in regard to etiology	Education
	  Consultation
	  Observation
		DCG

Criteria
  Client centered
  Singular
	Phases
	  Preparation
		Care plan revision
		  Nursing diagnoses

Observable
  Measurable
  Time limited
  Mutual
  Realistic
	Intervention
	  Communication
		Expected outcomes
		  Interventions
		
		Communication

APPENDICES

A

Head-to-Toe Assessment

OVERALL IMPRESSION

Level of consciousness: awake, lethargic, obtunded, comatose

General health status: good, fair, poor

Developmental: age, height, weight, physical maturity, psychologic maturity, grooming

Vital signs: temperature, pulses, respirations, blood pressure

Equipment: catheter, IV, O_2, tubes, monitor, wheel chair, etc.

HEAD

General: size, shape, symmetry, skin; edema, tenderness

Hair: amount, texture, cleanliness

Scalp: color, cleanliness, scaliness, lesions

Eyes: visual acuity, extraocular movement, pupils, iris, sclera, conjunctiva, eyelids; color, vascularity; discharge, lesions

Ears: auditory acuity, auricle, ear canal; lesions, discharge

Nose: olfactory acuity, septum, mucosa; lesions, discharge, congestion, flaring

Mouth: lips, gingiva, buccal mucosa, tongue, teeth, voice; symmetry, color, vascularity, lesions, hydration, odor; caries

NECK

Skin: color, vascularity; lesions

Pharynx: gag reflex, tonsils, color; inflammation, exudate

Trachea: deviation from midline

Thyroid: size, shape, symmetry; nodules

Lymph nodes: size, shape, mobility, delimitation; tenderness

Blood vessels: carotid arteries, jugular veins, pulse volume; distention

Range of motion: active, passive; pain, crepitation

THORAX

General: size, shape, symmetry, excursion; tenderness

Skin: color, vascularity, texture, turgor; lesions

Breasts: contour, symmetry, nipples; masses, discharge, tenderness

Axillae: nodes; lesions

Skeletal: spine, scapulae sternum, clavicles, ribs, alignment; deformities

Muscular: development, symmetry, strength; bulging, retractions, tenderness

Lungs: breathing patterns, lung sounds; cough, expectoration, fremitus, dullness to percussion

Heart: apical pulse patterns, valves, borders; murmurs, thrills

UPPER EXTREMITIES

General: size, proportion, symmetry, development, range of motion; tenderness

Skin: color, temperature; lesions

Pulses: radial, brachial; patterns, quality

Joints: symmetry, mobility; ankylosis, crepitation, swelling, tenderness

Muscles: symmetry, tone, strength, grips

Neurologic: sensation; paresthesias, tremors, spasms

Nails: color, capillary refill, grooming; clubbing, ridges

ABDOMEN

General: size, contour, symmetry; scars, pulsations, masses, tenderness, hernias
Skin: color, vascularity; lesions
Umbilicus: contour, location; protrusion
Sounds: normoactive, hyperactive, hypoactive, absent, aortic bruit
Liver: border location and regularity; lumps, tenderness
Stomach: gastric air bubble
Spleen: splenic dullness, palpability
Kidney: Palpability, tenderness; urinary output and characteristics
Bladder: distention, control
Bowel: regularity of output, characteristics

GENITALIA

General: development, color, vascularity; lesions, masses, discharge, odor
Male: penis, scrotum, testes
Female: labia majora, labia minora, urethral orifice, introitus

RECTUM

Skin: excoriation, lesions, hemorrhoids, tenderness, bleeding
Sphincter: muscle tone, control; nodules, tenderness

LOWER EXTREMITIES

General: size, proportion, symmetry, development, range of motion; tenderness

Skin: color, temperature; lesions

Vascular: femoral, popliteal, tibial, pedal pulses: rate, quality; warmth, color, perfusion; varicosities; Homan's sign

Joints: symmetry, mobility; ankylosis, crepitation, swelling, tenderness

Muscles: symmetry, tone, strength, gait

Neurologic: sensation; paresthesias, tremors, spasms

Nails: color, capillary refill, grooming; clubbing, ridges

Systems Assessment

OVERALL IMPRESSION

Appearance: age, sex, race, height, weight

NEUROLOGIC

Level of consciousness: awake, lethargic, obtunded, comatose

Sensory

Visual: acuity; pupil size, shape, equality, reaction to light, accommodation; extraocular movement; diplopia, photophobia, pain, burning; aids (glasses, contacts, prostheses)

Auditory: acuity; tinnitis, pain, vertigo; aids

Gustatory: salt, sweet, sour, bitter

Olfactory: ability of each nostril

Sensation: heat, cold, touch, pain; bilateral face, trunk, extremities; kinesthesia

Reflexes: superficial and deep tendon reflexes (DTRs), Babinski

RESPIRATORY

Nose: Nasal symmetry, mucosal color; congestion, flaring, edema, exudate, bleeding, lesions; sneezing, tenderness

Pharynx: mucosal color; spots, tenderness

Trachea: deviations, scars, tracheostomy

Chest: size, shape, symmetry, expansion; deformities, crepitation, retractions, use of accessory muscles, tactile fremitis, tenderness

Lungs: respiratory rate, regularity, depth; respiratory sounds: normal/adventitious, site, equality, intensity, quality, duration

CARDIAC

Apical pulse: rate, regularity, intensity, quality; murmurs

Heart: cardiac borders; thrills

VASCULAR

Arteries: pulse rates, quality; deficits, bruits

Veins: varicosities, jugular venous distention (JVD), tenderness

Capillaries: nail bed perfusion, refill; clubbing, cyanosis

Lymph: nodes: swelling, mobility, tenderness; edema

GASTROINTESTINAL

Mouth and throat: mucosal color, hydration; lesions, bleeding, edema; teeth: number, condition, dentures; tongue: symmetry, color, coating; gums: color; retraction; throat: gag reflex; tenderness, dysphagia

Abdomen: size, contour, symmetry, umbilicus, gastric air bubble, bowel sounds, liver border, splenic dullness; incision, scars, ostomy, masses, tenderness, guarding

Rectum: sphincter tone, control; excoriation, lesions, hemorrhoids, bleeding, tenderness

Digestion: eating patterns and habits; dyspepsia, postprandial discomfort

Elimination: regularity, quality, continence; constipation, diarrhea, discomfort; aids

RENAL

Kidneys: palpability; tenderness

Urine: output: quantity, quality, frequency, continence; dysuria

INTEGUMENTARY

Color: pink, pale, mottled, cyanotic, jaundiced, ruddy

Texture: turgor, dryness/oiliness, lesions (type, size, shape, color, distribution, discharge), masses (site, size, shape, mobility, tenderness)

MUSCULOSKELETAL

Muscles: size, symmetry, tone, strength; weakness, spasms, tremors

Bones: alignment; fractures

Joints: range of motion (active and passive); articular swelling, tenderness, rigidity, contractures, crepitation

Activity: level, frequency, ease

REPRODUCTIVE

Genitalia: color, odor, discharge, lesions, tenderness; males: penis, scrotum, testes; females: labia, urethral and vaginal orifices, menstruation

ENDOCRINE

Thyroid: goiter, exophthalmos

Pituitary: acromegaly/acromicria

Gonadal: sexual development for age

Metabolic: height/weight ratio, carbohydrate metabolism, fluid balance, electrolyte balance; metabolic disorders

HEMATOLOGIC

Erythrocytes: anemia, erythrocytosis; weakness, pallor
Leukocytes: leukopenia, leukocytosis; infection, fever
Thrombocytes: thrombocytopenia, thrombocytosis; petechiae, ecchymoses, bleeding, thromboses

PSYCHOSOCIAL

Mental status: oriented/disoriented, appearance, behavior, thought processes, cognitive functions, memory, mood, affect
Support system: family, friends, community
Coping ability: independent, interdependent, dependent

Client-Needs Assessment

OVERALL IMPRESSION

Level of assistance needed: total care; partial care; self-care education; social/community referrals

HEALTH PERCEPTION–HEALTH MANAGEMENT

Subjective: describe and compare: usual and current health status; symptoms, cause, and treatment for current illness; expectations for health status; compliance with previous therapy; anticipated self-care problems

Objective: assess and compare with client's perceptions: chronic and acute illnesses; knowledge about and self-care ability for illnesses and health maintenance; realism of health status expectations; motivation and ability to comply with prescribed therapy; self-care learning needs

NUTRITIONAL-METABOLIC

Subjective: describe and evaluate: usual and current daily food and fluid intake; appetite, eating, and digestion problems; understanding of and compliance with diet therapy; nutritional status, weight

Objective: assess and compare with client's perceptions: nutritional, fluid, and electrolyte status; food and fluid needs; actual food and fluid intake; gastrointestinal and metabolic function; potential nutritional, fluid, and electrolyte problems; nutritional knowledge and learning needs; motivation and ability to comply with prescribed therapies; self-care assistance needs

ELIMINATION

Subjective: describe and evaluate: bowel patterns, problems; urinary patterns, problems; skin condition, problems; understanding of and compliance with prescribed therapies

Objective: assess and compare with client's

perceptions: bowel output and function; renal output and function; skin condition; potential bowel, renal, and skin problems; elimination self-care knowledge and learning needs; motivation and ability to comply with prescribed therapy; self-care assistance needs

ACTIVITY-EXERCISE

Subjective: describe and evaluate: usual and current activity patterns; expectations for activity ability; self-care ability, problems, and expectations; compliance with prescribed activity level; actual and desired leisure activities

Objective: assess and compare with client's perceptions: activity level; functional motor ability, limitations; respiratory and cardiac status; activity tolerance, fatigue; self-care abilities and deficits; potential activity and self-care problems; understanding of prescribed exercises and learning needs; motivation and ability to comply with prescribed activities and exercises; assistive devices needed; community referrals needed; leisure activity ability and needs

SLEEP-REST

Subjective: describe and evaluate: usual and current sleep patterns; adequacy of rest; sleep problems, coping and sleep aids; expectations for sleep problem resolution

Objective: assess and compare with client's perceptions: sleep patterns, aids; energy level, mental status; environmental influences; potential sleep problems; sleep self-care learning needs

COGNITIVE-PERCEPTUAL

Subjective: describe and evaluate: mental abilities, memory; sensory deficits and aids; ability to cope with limitations; health care knowledge; discomforts, pain, and management; effectiveness of sensory therapies; expectations for resolution of sensory problems

Objective: assess and compare with client's perceptions: neurologic and mental status; sensory self-care ability; health care knowledge and learning needs; motivation and ability to comply with prescribed therapy; assistive devices needed; social/community referrals needed

SELF-PERCEPTION—SELF-CONCEPT

Subjective: describe and evaluate: body image; self-esteem; concerns, fears, anxieties; goals and expectations; effects of health status on self-image

Objective: assess and compare with client's perceptions: realism of body image, concerns, fears, expectations; emotional status; factors contributing to anxieties, self-concept problems; psychologic and emotional support needs; social support available; referral needs

ROLE-RELATIONSHIP

Subjective: describe and evaluate: roles: usual and current ability to fulfill and satisfaction with
relationships: independence-dependence
family: living arrangements, marital status, parenting, problems;
friends: availability, isolation;
community: participation, isolation;
communication: expressive and receptive adequacy

Objective: assess and compare with client's perceptions: roles and adequacy of ability to meet obligations; family and social support; communication abilities; personal, family counseling needs; community referral needs

SEXUALITY-REPRODUCTIVE

Subjective: describe and evaluate: usual and current sexual activity level; satisfaction with sexual life; effects of illness on sexuality and reproduction; self-care knowledge concerning sexual activity and reproduction; expectations for sexuality and reproduction

Objective: assess and compare with client's perceptions: sexual development for age, hormonal levels; sexual and reproductive self-care knowledge and learning needs; realism of sexual and reproductive expectations; sexual and reproductive counseling needs

COPING–STRESS TOLERANCE

Subjective: describe and evaluate: major life changes, stressors; decision-making ability; ability to cope with stress, stress management skills; stress management problems and needs

Objective: assess and compare with client's perceptions: vital signs, muscle tension, affect; level of anxiety; physiologic and emotional stressors; coping patterns; independence/dependence in decision making; knowledge of stress management skills and learning needs; social support; counseling needs

VALUE-BELIEF

Subjective: describe and evaluate: religious affiliation and satisfaction with; fundamental values, ethics, philosophy; effects of illness on beliefs; spiritual needs

Objective: assess and compare with client's perceptions: consistency of values and beliefs; degree of spiritual distress; spiritual counseling needs

B

**NORTH AMERICAN
NURSING DIAGNOSIS
ASSOCIATION
APPROVED NURSING
DIAGNOSTIC CATEGORIES**

EIGHTH CONFERENCE, 1988

PATTERN 1: EXCHANGING

Altered Nutrition: More than body requirements

Altered Nutrition: Less than body requirements

Altered Nutrition: Potential for more than body requirements

Potential for Infection

Potential Altered Body Temperature

Hypothermia

Hyperthermia

Ineffective Thermoregulation

Dysreflexia

Constipation
Perceived Constipation
Colonic Constipation
Diarrhea
Bowel Incontinence
Altered Patterns of Urinary Elimination
Stress Incontinence
Reflex Incontinence
Urge Incontinence
Functional Incontinence
Total Incontinence
Urinary Retention
Altered (specify type) Tissue Perfusion (renal, cerebral, cardiopulmonary, gastrointestinal, peripheral)
Fluid Volume Excess
Fluid Volume Deficit (1)
Fluid Volume Deficit (2)
Potential Fluid Volume Deficit
Decreased Cardiac Output
Impaired Gas Exchange
Ineffective Airway Clearance
Ineffective Breathing Pattern
Potential for Injury
Potential for Suffocation
Potential for Poisoning
Potential for Trauma
Potential for Aspiration

Potential for Disuse Syndrome
Impaired Tissue Integrity
Altered Oral Mucous Membrane
Impaired Skin Integrity
Potential Impaired Skin Integrity

PATTERN 2: COMMUNICATING

Impaired Verbal Communication

PATTERN 3: RELATING

Altered Family Processes
Altered Parenting
Potential Altered Parenting
Parental Role Conflict
Altered Role Performance
Sexual Dysfunction
Altered Sexuality Patterns
Social Isolation
Impaired Social Interaction

PATTERN 4: VALUING

Spiritual Distress (Distress of the Human Spirit)

PATTERN 5: CHOOSING

Impaired Adjustment
Ineffective Individual Coping
Defensive Coping

Family Coping: Potential for Growth
Ineffective Family Coping: Disabling
Ineffective Family Coping: Compromised
Decisional Conflict (specify)
Ineffective Denial
Health-Seeking Behaviors (specify)
Noncompliance (specify)

PATTERN 6: MOVING

Activity Intolerance
Potential Activity Intolerance
Altered Growth and Development
Altered Health Maintenance
Diversional Activity Deficit
Fatigue
Impaired Home Maintenance Management
Impaired Physical Mobility
Impaired Swallowing
Ineffective Breastfeeding
Bathing/Hygiene Self-Care Deficit
Dressing/Grooming Self-Care Deficit
Feeding Self-Care Deficit
Toileting Self-Care Deficit
Sleep Pattern Disturbance

PATTERN 7: PERCEIVING

Body-Image Disturbance
Self-Esteem Disturbance

Chronic Low Self-Esteem
Situational Low Self-Esteem
Personal Identify Disturbance
Hopelessness
Powerlessness
Sensory/Perceptual Alterations (specify):
  (visual, auditory, kinesthetic, gustatory,
  tactile, olfactory)
Unilateral Neglect

PATTERN 8: KNOWING

Altered Thought Processes
Knowledge Deficit (specify)

PATTERN 9: FEELING

Anxiety
Fear
Anticipatory Grieving
Dysfunctional Grieving
Pain
Chronic Pain
Potential for Violence: Self-directed or di-
  rected at others
Posttrauma Response
Rape–Trauma Syndrome
Rape–Trauma Syndrome: Compound Re-
  action
Rape–Trauma Syndrome: Silent Reaction

Glossary

actual That which exists. A problem that the client is currently experiencing. *See* Potential.

alleviate To ease, lessen, or relieve a symptom or a problem.

analysis The logical examination of and professional judgment about client data or problem status. Used in the diagnostic process to derive a nursing diagnosis and when SOAP charting to make a statement about the status of a problem.

assess To examine. To survey the biopsychosocial aspects of the client's status using professional knowledge and judgment. *See* Assessment.

assessment Examination of the client. Includes the interview, chart review, consultation, and physical examination, using the techniques of inspection, auscultation, palpation, and percussion. The first step of the nursing process; activities required in the first step are data collection, sorting, and documentation. The purpose is to gather information for health problem identification.

assistive care The level of nursing care in which the nurse and the client work together to perform health-care measures. The nurse supplements the client's capabilities, giving care only in areas in which the client is experiencing difficulty. The client is encouraged to do as much for himself or herself as is healthful.

augment To aid, support, magnify, add to, or potentiate.

care plan The written outline, or schema, that includes identification of the client's problems, goals for problem resolution, and specific interventions and nursing orders. The care plan documents and ensures use of the nursing process. A legal document that is part of the client's chart.

client centered A characteristic of a correctly written goal, specifying the client as the focus of the anticipated outcome.

collaboration The act of conferring or consulting with another for the purposes of gathering data, planning, implementing, and evaluating. Helps to maintain objectivity by adding another's viewpoint. Expands the data base and range of interventions by adding the consulted party's additional information and expertise. *See* Consultation.

congruency The agreement of harmony between two or more facts, pieces of data, or areas of assessment. An essential criterion in data validation.

consistency The agreement or conformity between the various parts of the assessment.

consultation The collaborative act of conferring with another, usually an expert in a particular field, for the purpose of obtaining skilled advice related to client care or services. *See* Collaboration.

criteria Standards, principles, or requirements established for accomplishing or evaluating an activity or condition.

criterion One norm, rule, or gauge for measuring the adequacy or validity of something. *See* Criteria.

data Facts, information. Usually categorized as subjective or objective. *See* Subjective and Objective.

datum One fact or piece of information. *See* Data.

dependent Those nursing actions that directly enact a physician's order and cannot be legally performed independently by the nurse but require nursing skill or expertise. Dependent nursing activities must always by guided by independent nursing assessment and judgment.

diagnosis A brief, formal statement that names a condition, situation, or problem, based on the professional assessment. *See* Nursing Diagnosis.

discharge goal The overall outcome anticipated for the client by the time of release from the medical institution. *See* Goal, Long-term Goal, Short-term Goal.

documentation All the entries in the client's medical record; these entries validate the client's problems and care and exist as a legal record.

education The teaching or instruction given to the client about health care and maintenance.

etiology The second part of the nursing diagnostic statement. That which affects, contributes to, or causes the problem. Directs the focus of nursing actions.

evaluate To appraise or judge. *See* Evaluation.

evaluation The professional appraisal or judgment of the effectiveness of nursing care. The fifth step of the nursing process during which a determination is made as to whether client goals were met. Requires reassessment of client status and may reactivate the entire nursing process.

goal The anticipated outcome of a client problem, stated in behavioral terms, that indicates resolution of the problem. Correctly written, goals are client centered, singular, observable, measurable, time limited, mutual, and realistic. *See* Discharge Goal, Long-term Goal, Short-term Goal.

health-care team All those people, departments, and ancillary services that collectively render care and services to the client.

implement To carry out a proposed plan; to use the care plan in client care delivery. *See* Implementation.

implementation The actual application of the care plan during client care delivery. The fourth step of the nursing process. Involves preparation, actual nursing care as planned, and documentation of the client's responses to the interventions. *See* Implement.

independent Autonomous nursing actions that are legally performed by virtue of the nurse's education and license and the role of nursing itself. Not dependent on another's authority.

interdependent Collaborative nursing actions that require another professional's expertise or that depend on a medical order to initiate.

intervention A specific nursing action that is carried out to restore, maintain, or promote the client's health. Nursing treatments given during the implementation step of the nursing process.

interview An organized, systematic conversation with the client designed to obtain pertinent health-related subjective information.

long-term goal The anticipated outcome of the client's problem, as identified in the problem portion of the nursing diagnosis statement. A statement in behavioral terms indicating resolution of the client problem. *See* Goal, Discharge Goal, Short-Term Goal.

management A type of nursing intervention that includes all nursing technologies and physical care measures.

measurable A characteristic of a correctly written goal, specifying that the anticipated change in behavior or status is quantifiable by some means.

narrative charting The method of charting usually used in the source-oriented method of record keeping. A prose description of the client's status and activity. *See* SOAP Charting, Source-Oriented Medical Record.

nursing diagnosis The formal statement of an actual or potential health problem that nurses can legally and independently treat. The second step of the nursing process during which the client's actual and potential unhealthful responses to an illness or condition are identified. Requires professional analysis and interpretation of the data gathered during the assessment.

nursing orders An intervention statement written by the nurse that is within the independent role of nursing to plan and initiate.

nursing process The systematic, logical, problem-solving method by which nurses individualize care for each client. The five steps of the nursing process are assessment, diagnosis, planning, implementation, and evaluation.

objective Information that can be observed by others; free of feelings, perceptions, prejudices.

observable That which can be perceived and validated. All objective data are observable. Also a criterion for goal-setting; the desired outcome must be able to be detected by another.

observation That which is noticed or perceived by any of the senses. Does not include those subjective experiences of the client that cannot be verified or validated by another person. *See* Observable. Also a type of nursing intervention in which the client's status and response to nursing care is assessed.

quality assurance A system of auditing client care and medical records for the purposes of establishing, assuring, and maintaining high standards of client care delivery.

plan The systematic design of an organized method for client care delivery and meeting the client's identified needs. Includes setting goals, devising appropriate interventions, and documenting the care plan on the client's chart. The third step of the nursing process.

POMR Problem-oriented medical record. A system of record keeping and documentation that focuses on the client's health-related problems and a health-care team approach to client care. The medical record has four sections: data base, problem list, care plan, and progress notes. All members of the health-care team use the same sections. *See* Source-Oriented Medical Record.

potential A status placed before a nursing diagnosis statement when the problem does not yet actually exist but is likely to occur unless preventive action is taken. Written when high-risk factors associated with the problem exist. *See* Actual.

psychosocial A type of nursing intervention that deals with the client's mental, emotional, and social concerns.

realistic A characteristic of a correctly written goal, specifying that the anticipated change in behavior or status be practical and achievable.

referral The recommendation that the client see an expert for the purposes of gaining information or assistance.

short-term goal The anticipated outcome, stated in behavioral terms, that indicates alleviation or resolution of the etiology portion of the nursing diagnosis statement. *See* Goal, Discharge Goal, Long-Term Goal.

significant other(s) Those persons who are closest to, intimately involved with, and important to the client; usually family members and close friends.

singular A characteristic of a correctly written goal, specifying that the outcome name only one anticipated change in behavior or status.

SOAP charting The method of writing progress notes

when using the problem-oriented medical record system. Progress notes focus on an identified problem and include the client's subjective perceptions, the health-care team member's objective observations, an analysis of the current status of the problem, and a plan statement. *See* Narrative Charting, POMR.

source-oriented medical record A system of record keeping and documentation in which the client's chart is divided into sections corresponding to the various components of the health-care team. *See* POMR.

subjective Information gathered from client statements; the client's feelings and perceptions. Not verifiable by another except by inference.

supportive care The level of nursing care in which the nurse provides information and encouragement to the client who is capable of performing self-care measures.

time limited A characteristic of a correctly written goal, specifying that the anticipated change in behavior or status be accomplished in a definite time period.

total care The level of nursing care in which the nurse performs all activities for the client, who is completely incapacitated.

validate To confirm, verify, or corroborate the accuracy of assessment data or the appropriateness of the care plan.

INDEX